EPIDEMIC
OF
COURAGE

EPIDEMIC OF COURAGE

Facing AIDS in America

Lon G. Nungesser

St. Martin's Press / New York

EPIDEMIC OF COURAGE.
Copyright © 1986 by Lon G. Nungesser.
All rights reserved.
Printed in the United States of America.
No part of this book may be used or reproduced
in any manner whatsoever without written permission
except in the case of brief quotations
embodied in critical articles or reviews.
For information, address St. Martin's Press,
175 Fifth Avenue, New York, N.Y. 10010.

Design by M. Paul

Library of Congress Cataloging in Publication Data

Nungesser, Lon G.
    Epidemic of Courage.

    1. AIDS (Disease)--United States--Psychological
aspects.   2. AIDS (Disease)--United States--Social
aspects.   I. Title.
RC607 .A26N86   1986   362.1'969792   85-25087
ISBN 0-312-25751-1

First Edition

10 9 8 7 6 5 4 3 2 1

This book is dedicated to the virtues of faith, hope, love, and compassion.

Contents

Acknowledgments

I am grateful to the people who shared their thoughts, feelings, and desires with me. Thanks to my friends and family for the support needed to be so involved with the AIDS health crisis. Special thanks go to Bill, whose steadfast love gave me the strength to stand strong in the face of cynicism and adversity. I acknowledge the editorial assistance of Carolyn Estey. I thank Bobby Reynolds for his invaluable assistance. Thanks to Philip Zimbardo and Rosanne S. for their concern and encouragement.

Foreword

Lon G. Nungesser's book gathers astonishing raw energy as it focuses sharply and relentlessly on the devastating AIDS epidemic that is causing not only medical but also emotional and spiritual havoc among ever increasing numbers in our country.

The author, who has AIDS himself, has interviewed both people with AIDS and those who are deeply involved and concerned with this crisis. The resulting discussions are uncompromising when it comes to the expression of personal opinions, which are rough-hewn, always candid and arresting. The interviews are edifying, consciousness-raising, and informative.

"This crisis has put purpose back into a lot of people's lives, especially people who died and people who are serving people who are dying," says a New York man who has known nearly nine hundred people with AIDS.

One San Francisco man who has AIDS declares: "Gay men are strong men—especially emotionally . . . and are not afraid to hug and hold on to one another in crisis. . . . Perhaps we have already been an example to those who do not understand our sexual persuasion. At least they can see the love we have for each other as people."

A lesbian psychotherapist in California remembers fondly a gay colleague and close friend who died of AIDS. "By being himself, he brought out the soft side in people who would ordinarily just not let that out. So, he just *was* love, you know?

And by being who he was—and he moved into that more and more—he was transformed and he transformed other people."

How, in her view, has AIDS affected the gay male community?

"Its sobering effect has resulted in more cohesiveness, more caring, and more genuine emotional expression toward one another. It's as though the community were in its adolescence before and is now painfully entering manhood."

Support people in the AIDS crisis appear many times in the pages of this book. One, a counseling coordinator working with AIDS patients, describes to Nungesser how she let go of her ego and her preconceptions. "I think I've learned to live with uncertainty. . . . Learning to be a good follower in a dance where the music changes rapidly. . . . I've given up looking at or worrying about the future. I think I'm more in the moment than I've ever been."

And, she expresses a thought ineffably touching: "I wish we could all be as loving as so many of the gay brothers have been to their friends dying—to everyone. There would be world peace."

The special gift of this book is its absence of phoniness. It contains rage, passion, bitterness, and unpopular views as well as tenderness, quiet simplicity, gentle warmth, and the expression of genuine diversity. To read it is to share an illuminating experience of courage in living, dying, and loving.

—*Malcolm Boyd*

Preface

This is a book of interviews with people whose lives have been affected by AIDS. I have a very personal involvement in the subject of this book; I have the disease myself. To write this book I have marshaled all my abilities and skills, my knowledge and adaptability. Each of us must take responsibility for facing this illness and fashioning our own response to this social crisis. I seek information about my illness and make decisions about quality care. I strive to survive. When I need, I seek to meet the need. If my environment is not supportive, I challenge, change, or otherwise cope with it. I view myself as a writer and a psychologist, not a diseased homosexual.

Whatever my life brings, I feel confident I can experience it. That is all I really require of myself—honest experience followed by honest expression. The hope that drives me is the desire to fully complete my contribution of love to and for humanity. To reveal the reality of AIDS as one who is living through it is the contribution I have to offer.

Introduction

Acquired Immune Deficiency Syndrome (AIDS) may be the biological mystery of our time, but one certainty burns amid medical mayhem: People around the globe are besieged by the *psychological* crisis of AIDS. Strategies for coping with chronic life-threatening illness range from dealing with the illness head-on to retreating from it. Some people with AIDS believe they will die soon; they may become helpless and hopeless. Others believe that treatments for AIDS symptoms are more deadly than the disease itself; they may become helpful to others who are dealing with AIDS and to themselves. Some people believe that AIDS is caused by God's wrath and may say "Let 'em die." Still others believe that AIDS is the product of biological warfare or that it is an iatrogenic epidemic (a widespread disease caused by medical treatment). These beliefs shape one's entire psychological reaction to AIDS, persons with AIDS, and AIDS health and human services. The day-to-day quality of life for persons with AIDS is determined by their ever-changing ways of coping with the chronic stresses of AIDS.

The purpose of *Epidemic of Courage* is to portray the psychological experience of people during the evolving AIDS epidemic. The interviews in this book, conducted between February and October of 1984, reveal what one may do to adapt to this health crisis. Actions that increase the quality of life for people who have an indeterminate amount of time are encouraged. Tales of heroes facing insurmountable challenges with courage and wisdom are told. *Epidemic of Courage* documents the hopes and visions of young men facing death at an early age.

PART ONE

Persons with Aids

1

A Multicolored Mosaic

Arthur Felson

Arthur Felson is a forty-year-old gay man with CDC-defined AIDS. He has toxoplasmosis. He lives in New York City and works as a full-time health advocate. Before his illness he was a newspaper reporter, writer, and publisher.

I

Artie, when did you first become aware of the emerging AIDS crisis?

'77.

Where did you learn of this?

Through a friend of mine who had already come down with it. He had all of the symptoms, including lesions. He eventually had to have one of his limbs amputated. From what I understood, he had severe meningitis and then cerebral dysfunction. That was my first contact with a person with AIDS.

There was no information in '77. There was no medical

information at all. I saw a friend of mine die. I remember him running around from one hospital to the other, not really getting very much of an answer. They weren't telling him what he had. He was seeing one of what turned out to be the best doctors, and they knew a bit. They knew his immune system was impaired. They knew that he had cancer, but by and large, that's all that was known.

So you were pretty much aware as soon as the term *GRID* [Gay Related Immune Deficiency] came out?

Oh, yes, I was involved. In fact, I was diagnosed as having GRID in 1979.

And then you were diagnosed as having AIDS after that?

Yes, the CDC [Center for Disease Control] diagnosed me with AIDS. I was involved in the original case control cluster study.

How many people do you know right now who have AIDS?

I only know about three people that don't. In terms of close personal friends, I would say well over a hundred. To many of them, I'm very close.

What illnesses and stages of the illnesses do these persons with AIDS [PWAs] have?

They go the complete gamut from people who may—who are fearful that they're going to come down with it, through people who were diagnosed around the same time as I was and progressed all the way through KS [Kaposi's sarcoma] and

PCP [Pneumocystis carinii pneumonia]. Some people have died.

When did you first notice a warning sign, like a lymph node swelling?

In '78 I started having night sweats.

What were your presenting symptoms when you were diagnosed?

Low-grade fevers, generalized lymphadenopathy, and thrush. Weight loss—*massive* weight loss: fifty pounds! Pain, unexplained pain in my limbs, headaches, nausea, and unexplained diarrhea for seven months. I had every one of those symptoms.

Was your experience of the illness what you expected?

Yes and no. I didn't die. I expected to. I expected everyone that had the illness to die. I didn't expect myself to come through this, okay? Yet, it wasn't the worst experience of my life. Dealing with people who did die certainly *was* the worst experience. The illness itself has been a real pain in the ass. But I felt that, for me, I could deal with it. I think I've been lucky. In many ways, I think I've been lucky.

What is your perception of the ways others have reacted to you?

Initially, I would say, up to the last two years, people have been real, real nice. I'm talking about everyone I come into contact with. The last two years have been very hard because I've been very public, and I've gotten a lot of rejection from that.

To some degree I think it's their own denial, their own failure to take responsibility in their own life-styles. Looking at the way I've started taking responsibility in my life-style, they're not able to deal with it. I think, to some degree, one of my family members was afraid. A lot of people fear that they can casually contract the disease.

I think some people now have seen me become public and are more concerned about my gayness than they are about my AIDS.

How do you think you caught AIDS, and how do you think other people may catch AIDS?

That's a hard question for me to answer. Let me deal with the second half of it. I think that there is an epidemic that is going on in the gay community; if people continue to put themselves into positions that present risks to themselves, then I think the possibilities are very severe for our community. The risks are well known. They range from dietary and stress factors through continuation of certain kinds of sexual activities that may put them in health crisis.

In terms of how I caught—or how I perceive that I caught AIDS, there were activities I was doing prior to '78 that were injurious to my health, that seem to have played a role in the development of AIDS. It's because of those activities that I believe I came down with the illness. I don't believe I came down with the illness solely because I was a sexually active man. I believe I came down with the illness because I was a highly stressed, drug-abusing, sexually active man who was nutritionally insufficient and who was psychologically insufficient. I may have had a minimum amount of genetic predisposition.

How do you think, for yourself right now, that you're at risk of catching other opportunistic infections?

Luck.

How would you define risky sex?

Well, I wouldn't define anything as *risky* sex, because
that's judgmental. I think that people take risks in everything
they do. I mean, if a person, for example, is barely meeting
their nutritional standards, and is working in a high-stress environment, doing lots of cocaine, the chances for them to come
down with a heart attack are much better than an individual
who's exercising, not doing drugs, dealing with stress, and
dealing with nutrition in a proper way. So there are risky
things that we do, but in terms of sexual activity, I think people had better start being a little bit more careful in the way
that they look at their own sexuality, particularly gay men, and
in the way that they make determinations on what other people *should* do.

So these definitions of safe sex and risky sex—

I don't buy it. And the reason I don't buy it is, number
one, we have to constantly affirm our gayness. By that I mean,
in a time of epidemic, to totally stop having sex is, for me,
going back into the closet. There are kinds of sexual activities
that can make sex, not necessarily safer, but healthier. Using
condoms, for example, may cut down the spread of STDs
[sexually transmitted diseases]. From what I understand, vi-
ruses have a difficult time passing through condom mem-
branes. So, in terms of gonorrhea and syphilis, that will make
sex healthier. Rimming is a dangerous sexual practice today
because of the epidemic of amebiasis. So, sex would be
healthier if people didn't rim.

People talk about "sexual compulsivity." That's bullshit.
That's psychobabble. People need to do everything in modera-

tion. And people must make their own judgments about what the definition of moderation is for them. I don't think people can say that other people are sexually compulsive in the same way that you can say that people who eat a lot are compulsive. There is no similarity.

I think *safer sex* is a good key word that has come about primarily as a result of Michael Callen's work here in New York City. But it is only a key word. I think what Michael is *really* going after is not *safer sex*, but a *healthier sexual conduct:* a sense of ethical and personal responsibility in sex. People get lined up on either side of the battle only because of the key word. When you hear *safer sex*, you automatically think there is "unsafe sex." Well, there's healthy sex and there's unhealthy sex, and we're talking about AIDS as a health issue and eventually talking about sex as a health issue.

How do you think the government should prevent AIDS from spreading?

Well, the first thing that the government should do is to take AIDS out of a political atmosphere in terms of a research issue. And I don't think that's going to happen with a Republican president. Secondly, the amount of research being conducted on AIDS is questionable. The government refuses to tell private individuals or the general public what it's spending its money on. We don't know, for example, whether the government is spending *any* money on the development of an LAV virus vaccine. We know that they're working on HTLV-III. But HTLV-III may not be the same as LAV.

So, we don't know what research is being done. The government's educational program is nonexistent. Have *you* seen—let me ask this question rhetorically—anything put out by the government on AIDS and gay male sexuality?

Well, they put out a little two-year-old booklet on AIDS

and gay men that was obviously not written by a gay person. What we're seeing is a heterosexualist health establishment trying to tell gay men how to live their lives. That spells a death knell to anything that comes out of Washington. (Coughs).

Okay, I'm going to shift gears and ask about some of your reactions to AIDS itself. How has the AIDS crisis made you feel?

It makes me feel, on one hand, incredible anger and, on the other hand, incredible numbness. But I would say, overall, that it has renewed in me the desire to live.

How did it do that?

By seeing so many people in so many different ways struggling in a day-to-day situation, in an hour-to-hour situation, to fight off the oppressions of death and disease and politics and everything else only for one thing, and that is to live—that has served as a challenge for me to live.

What about your desire to live in 1978?

I wouldn't say it was too good. I was living for the moment and not living for tomorrow.

Have you noticed a lot of changes in your gay identity?

Every aspect of my personality has changed. I no longer believe that being gay means having sex. Being gay is much, much more. It's culture, it's history, it's romanticism, it's caring. It is a life-style, and life is the first part of that style.

What is your perception of society's reaction to the AIDS epidemic?

As a journalist who worked the mainstream of society, and now being the person who's being reported on outside of the mainstream of society, I can understand a lot about what other people have struggled for and are struggling for. It's astounding to feel like a minority. It's astounding to be at the other end of being discriminated against. It's astounding to see the degree of irresponsibility that exists among people who are in what should be responsible positions. Having gone through the AIDS hysteria sweep and then having gone through the rush for information, and now going through what I call a nationwide AIDS-denial phase, I'm astounded that responsibility has not been as forthcoming in the straight community as it has in the gay community.

I think the gay and lesbian community have done something for themselves that the straight community hasn't even touched. We have evolved a system of health care for our people that is effective and is working. It involves large numbers of people and it serves as a model for what establishment health care could be.

I have to stress it's not only a gay male model. I mean, lesbians in America have done something that they should be proud of. They have brought community a step further. The number of women—gay women—involved in AIDS work is phenomenal. What they're doing across the country, whether it's a blood drive in Los Angeles—donating blood for gay men in Los Angeles—or fundraising or answering phones in Boston, or reaching out to break down the barriers of discrimination in hospitals in New York by working within the system, they have played a role.

What kinds of emotions have you experienced in response to your loved ones who have had AIDS or who have died of AIDS?

My lover committed suicide a year and a half ago.

Oh, I'm sorry. (Pause.) Did he have AIDS?

No. He was afraid he was going to come down with it. So my emotions have been very massive in terms of how I felt about him, my family, and my gay nuclear family. I think I'm better today and my family is healthier today and I'm closer with my gay and straight family today than I was a year and a half ago.

I hope that people were very supportive of you during that time.

Some were; some weren't. I mean, some people could deal with it and other people couldn't. Some people tend to look at the worst side, the side of death and of people with lesions and losing hair and say, "Oh, my God, isn't this terrible!" But there's another side. There's a side of getting to know someone who looks very different and getting to know an inner beauty that far surpasses a person's external appearance. Of getting to be close with people who really are living and who are over-coming illness as best they can, who function despite every-thing, who are able to walk around despite pain, who are disfigured, who were told that they wouldn't live very long and yet are, and who are trying experimental things, ah, who are human guinea pigs; I mean, these are people who should be positive examples to other people. And you don't read those stories. You don't see that in *Time* magazine, and you don't see that in the *Bay Area Reporter*, and you don't see that on NBC.

I mean, the guy at the Olympics the other day is a good example. I'm doing a newsletter for GMHC [Gay Men's Health Crisis] called *Winning*; it took a lot of persuasion to get them to back this project. We've already come out with one edition and we'll be coming out with one every month. But the objective is to tell good stories. People need hope. And they accepted that idea. One story I'm working on is this U.S. Gold Greco-Roman wrestler who had Hodgkin's disease! He had his spleen removed! He was on chemotherapy for nine and a half months! And came back to the Olympics and won the Gold.

That's fantastic!

That's the kind of stories to tell. I mean, when a guy's home and feeling real shit and is reaching out, okay, for someone to give him a glimpse of hope, and the doctors are telling him, "Well, we're going to put you on VP16 and you're going to feel like shit, and get a will done," and GMHC sends over a person to do their will! I mean, they want to hear something positive. They want to have some hope for the future.

What one word best describes your feelings about AIDS?

Hope.

II

Do you recall a time in which you became ill with a cold or some other seemingly common illness before you were told you had GRID?

I started losing energy two years before I went to the doctor. I kept going to the doctor expecting to get a positive result to a mononucleosis test. I had come down with every illness in the book before I got a diagnosis of GRID. I had hepatitis, I had gonorrhea, I had syphilis, I had herpes, I had nonspecific urethritis, specific urethritis, colds, allergies. I mean, every illness possible!

What was the most alarming symptom you had, that really led you to go in and get diagnosed?

Oh, I have to say my energy loss. It was massive. In '76, around the time of the bicentennial, I was full of energy. By '78 I was taking naps at work.

Did you feel like a victim of misfortune?

Not after three and a half hours' worth of questions by two CDC doctors. After listening to the way he was asking them, the kinds of questions, and his reactions to the questions, reactions to the answers, I realized that the government knew less than what gay doctors knew. And here I was, at that point, the victim, okay, and *I* knew more answers than both of them!

(Laughs.) I'm not surprised.

Okay. And at that point I said, "They're telling me that I'm going to die and they don't know half the answers to the questions that I do." So at that point I said, "You're on your own, kid." At that point my whole attitude changed. I no longer felt the victim, I no longer felt the patient.

What year was this?

I'd say this was '80.

What kind of changes in your economic and social life did all this bring about?

When your whole phone book dies, your social system breaks up. Economics? I was making a lot of money—a *lot* of money. Okay. I can't find a job in an *AIDS* organization, much less in a straight organization. And I'm one of about ten of the most vocal people in America today. My résumé, theoretically, should make me acceptable to anyone, and I cannot find work.

After some time passed since your diagnosis, did you take stock and reevaluate your life?

Yes. I started taking more responsibility for my life. I started being more particular about my food intake. I've now started to look at my body and started to exercise a little bit. I have totally changed my dating pattern. Since I don't drink, I don't go to gay bars. Since I'm looking for a relationship, I think all people are looking for relationships in one way or another, I'm now starting to have to talk to more people. And that is new to me. Before my diagnosis, it was easy for me to go to bed with someone and *then* get to know them. I no longer do that. I don't abuse my body any longer, which is a major step. I've become closer with my family, particularly with my parents, as I see them growing much older and going through their own health crises. AIDS has made me a little bit more able to deal more responsibly with them. I understand what it's like to be in a hospital. I understand what it's like to be on a ventilator. I understand what it's like to be concerned about not having enough money to buy medicine. So I can understand more of what they're experiencing. That has brought us together.

Did you feel like you deserved the illness?

That's judgmental. Before diagnosis, I wasn't judgmental. During diagnosis, I wasn't judgmental. After diagnosis, my intellect kept playing a role that oftentimes ran into opposition with my emotions. I mean, you have to understand that what's going on is that I would—well, you do understand. I mean, you do know. Sometimes I have to apologize, because I slip out and forget that you are involved also.

Yeah, very. (Laughs.)

Okay. So understand that sometimes I forget that.

That's all right, because I know how you feel. I mean, it's not very often that you get interviewed by somebody who has AIDS and who—well, I'm right in the middle of it.

What I find is, at times my emotions, okay, run into conflict with my intellect. If I listen to my intellect, it'll work out better than if I listen to my emotions.

How do you make sense out of the illness? And during this period of taking stock and reevaluating, what'd you come up with?

It's a growth thing. It's another part of life. Nobody gives us a piece of paper at birth that says, "Hey, it's going to be rosy for the rest of your life."

I didn't expect ever to come down with a disease that at the age of forty would make me start questioning how long I was going to be here. I didn't expect to cry as much as I have. I didn't expect *ever, ever* to—to lose as many people as I have. But it's happening. And through each experience, through every time I go to a funeral, I come out stronger. Every time I lose someone, I learn something. I learn something about myself, I learn something about other people. So the one thing that's happened that has been totally unexpected is that I've grown. And I think I've mellowed, I think I've become much more human, I think I've become much more aware, and I know I've become much more caring.

Have your needs for intimacy changed?

I've become an eighteenth-century romantic. I've become much more honest and up-front, and when I need to be nourished, I now have friends who will hold me. There are people I now have met who I can sleep with. Sex is marvelous. I've become very outspoken about it, and it's ironic that the more that I publicly talk about sexuality, the less sex I actually have! I don't know why that happens, but it's been happening that way. Sex is—again—a key word. And it's real volatile.

Well, you have not had KS, right?

No. Was the concern that the sex partner is going to see a lesion? If that's what you're asking, I've got an answer for it.

That's not what I was going to ask, but go ahead and give me the answer.

The answer is, when you've gone through massive weight loss and you look like a skeleton that's just come out of Auschwitz, the reaction is the exact same as when a person sees a lesion. You have a responsibility to inform the person before you have sex, no matter what kind of sexual activity it is, that you have AIDS. That deals with the subject immediately. You've already explained what's going on, so you don't have to worry about the lesion or weight loss. Some people will freak and say, "I can't have sex with you. It's immoral for you to even discuss it with me." Other people will go, "Let's immediately hop into bed because it's something new and different." And other people will be genuine and caring and—and touching.

Have your beliefs about gay freedom changed any since you became aware of AIDS?

I believe that gay freedom is just that: freedom to be gay, in every way possible. Freedom for a gay man to be able to go anywhere in America. Freedom for a gay woman to do anything that she's capable of doing. I think the worst thing that can happen is for us to start classifying ourselves. The worst thing that can happen is for an AIDS organization to say, "You can't come into this support group, because this support group is only for KS people." A gay man with KS being told, "You can't drink in a gay bar because you're going to infect the glasses." Or a gay man from San Francisco being told, "You cannot come into a gay bathhouse in New York City."

What is your impression about the bathhouse issue in San Francisco?

My impression about the bathhouse situation anywhere is that anyone should be able to go anywhere in America today.

Has this changed your beliefs about democracy in America?

It has. I'm much more cynical. I'm very concerned—and now we're going to get into it a little bit—*very* concerned about the self-righteous attitude that a great many people who are gay have about the sexual aspects of people who have AIDS. People would like us to be asexual. People would like us to go back into the closet. And people would like us to become victims. There are health problems at bathhouses, but until someone comes up with a way in which gay men can affirm their gayness, can see other gay men without their clothes on, without fear of being beaten up or robbed, then there *is* no alternative. Are we suggesting that gay men, in order to meet their sexual needs, become alcoholics? Are we suggesting that people pay a fee to meet people? I don't buy this. I really don't, and one of the problems that I constantly run up against is people saying, "Well, we have an epidemic that kills people. Therefore, people who have AIDS should be asexual. Otherwise they're being part of the process that kills people." I can't believe that. And I hear that from people who have AIDS.

Have your values about life and death changed any?

Well, I work to live. I mean, living takes a lot of work. Quality living takes a lot of work. And death is just a transition. Ah, I'm not afraid of it. In fact, if it comes, it might even be enjoyable. No one who's died has come back to complain.

I want to shift gears again here, and ask you a few questions. How do you think mainstream medicine has reacted to this?

If there is ever to be an indictment, it's going to be about mainstream medicine. There are many good, competent physicians, gay and straight, in America today. But it is a crime that it took so long for so little to have happened. There are at least 100,000 cases of AIDS in America today.

How does mainstream medicine relate to government control of AIDS?

Mainstream medicine *is* government control.

What do you think would be a more effective relationship between health care and government?

Nothing positive can happen between that tripart figure of gay medicine, mainstream medicine, and government until government and mainstream medicine recognize the specific and necessary role of gay medicine. There are no training facili-

ties for gay physicians as gay physicians in mainstream medicine. Gay medicine is not recognized as a distinctive medical
subspecialty.

**What about alternative medicine, homeopathic medicine?
Has it fared any better in treating people with AIDS?**

It's fared obviously worse in terms of other people's perception of its effectiveness. However, I think what we are now
seeing, thanks in a great deal to many people who have AIDS,
is a greater and greater recognition that a combined role may
be the ultimate answer in medicine today. A joining together
of established medical procedures and established Western
medicine working with alternative medical treatments and alternative medical disciplines may be the best mode of medicine. When you can take holistic health care and guided
visualization and homeopathic medical treatments and all
kinds of very valuable, longtime medical modalities established
in many other cultures, and combine that with some of the
best features of Western medicine, then we may have an op-
timal system of medicine. But that's only one part, because
then we have to have that system available for delivery to the
masses.

All people must recognize that the doctor is not a god, and
that the doctor doesn't have all the answers, and that medicine
and health care have to stress as much the prevention as the
treatment. Otherwise, we're not going to have a medical system that's humanistic. And that's our long-range goal. Human-
ism in medical care is what's coming out of AIDS. We're
teaching people to be compassionate, and we're teaching physicians to be compassionate.

What other long-term positive outcomes might there be?

Well, we're starting to see some symbols of them. The

Community Health Project here in New York has been a long time in coming. The Community Center here in New York, which is a multiservice, primary health-care facility—I mean, New York is New York, and it has not had one until now. I think that's a step forward. I think the growth of the National Lesbian and Gay Health Education Foundation is another example. The growth of Physicians for Human Rights chapters across the country, which has proliferated in the last five years, is an example.

There are all kinds of things starting to happen in the overall picture that can be looked at: GMHC, the AIDS/KS Foundation in San Francisco, support groups, hotlines. These can be looked at in the long-range view of being supportive services for gay men and lesbians. These supportive services set the role and a model for the mainstream health society.

So I think that the long-range objectives are starting to be looked at, are starting to be addressed, but there are many challenges, and we have to remember that AIDS is only one of those challenges. I mean, just take a look, for example, at aging. Our population is aging. There are more gay people who are older today than there were ten years ago. As the overall population increases, we're going to have to start thinking about gay nursing homes. We're going to have to start thinking about gay retirement centers. We're going to start having to think about subsidized health care for our gay senior citizens. And what's going to happen, as we've seen in AIDS, is we're going to have to take care of our own. We cannot rely upon government to give out a $200 check each month and say that's enough for our senior citizens to live on.

Tell me, Artie, if you could paint the history of this yourself, how would you have the AIDS epidemic be remembered?

As a mosaic. As being a mosaic of different colors going—

including blacks, okay, and I don't mean in terms of race. Think of a painting. It would be a mosaic of different colors. AIDS has shown me that we're very different, but we have a great deal in common. It's a common thread. We have a quilt, we have a patchwork, okay, and it's very well knit, and sometimes people die.

But there are a lot of people with a lot of life in them, and, I don't know, maybe I'm just overcompensating, but I see a lot of people every day who are *not* dying. Even the few that are in their death process are learning about living. That makes things much more hopeful. It gives me a hope for the future, and, ah, if I come down with KS tomorrow or pneumocystis tomorrow, I can say to myself, I've done something, and I'm content.

Sure, I get sad, I get depressed. I get disillusioned at times, and I lose my way; but something in the end brings it back. I think it's a lot to do with the courage of so many people around me.

Well, you're pretty strong inside yourself; I can tell just from talking to you this little bit.

Yeah, it comes. The strength comes after you see your first real close friend die.

Yes, of course. Someone once told me when I was a kid, if you were a piece of wood and a bowl was being carved out of you, it would hurt like hell, but you'd be able to hold all sorts of wonderful things.

And once it's seasoned—once that bowl is seasoned, it becomes a work of art.

Yeah. Well, it sounds like that's where we're at, and

maybe it's not all that bad, really. Of course, it's got its terrible parts.

You know what it is? We almost expect people to be obliged to say that AIDS is the worst thing in their life. If someone says, "It isn't so bad," or "It isn't the worst thing in my life," or that "It may have been the best thing in my life," it's almost as bad as people—people expect you to feel guilty for saying that. And you get other people who have AIDS who say to you, "Don't say that." (They laugh.) "Don't say that." I mean—or people will say, "Well, he's burned out." That's garbage. I mean, there are a lot of negative events. Who wants someone to die? I mean, we don't want that to happen. But the Indians were right. The Indians were right. When people die, they move on. The process doesn't necessarily have to be terrible. Get your tribe together, and you let the person die. And you help them to die, okay? *Give them the strength to die!*

And you get the tribe together. I like that.

They certainly seem to have had at least part of the answer, as far as I'm concerned.

It isn't all that bad. It's painful, it's a *noodge*, it's a pain in the *tuchas!* Hey, I mean, I'd prefer being a bodybuilder!

2

The Problem Is No Control

Bob Cecchi

Bob Cecchi is a forty-two-year-old gay man living on Manhattan's Upper West Side. He has some of the signs of AIDS, but has not been diagnosed as CDC-defined AIDS. Therefore, he is in the "gray zone." Bob was a carpenter before his diagnosis with Gay Related Immune Deficiency. He was on the Board of the New York Gay Men's Health Crisis when I spoke with him. (He knows nearly 900 persons with AIDS, representing all risk groups.) His comments about the problems of persons with AIDS are enlightening.

I

What is your occupation now?

Well, what I do for work right now is work for the Gay Men's Health Crisis. It's a volunteer job. I've been there two years. I don't get paid.

What do you do for them?

Up until last week I was assistant director of clinical services. Someone has been given a paid job with more credentials than I have, so they've taken that title. I probably will end up being patient ombudsman, which is the line of work that I'm doing and the new job is just a public acknowledgment of that.

What's a typical day for you?

A typical day for me is going into the office around ten, working until about eight or nine at night. Most of the time I am on the phone dealing with newly diagnosed people, ah, giving them—a kind of hope that they have not heard in the time it's taken them to be diagnosed and all that kind of stuff.

How many intakes do you do in a day?

I don't actually do what we call an intake. That's done by mental health professionals who go out to see a client, but, in a normal day's time, I might talk to maybe five patients, maybe five or six crisis counselors or buddies, maybe two social workers from the various hospitals, sometimes the Commission on Human Rights, maybe GMHC's lawyer, spend some time with the Financial Aid Department, and a part of the day is spent in conversation or consultation or supervision with the clinical director, the intake coordinator, you know, and we exchange ideas about what we think is going on with a certain client. It's basically an interesting day. It's also sometimes just extremely difficult. We had four patients die in the last two days. So today I spent the afternoon at a requiem mass for an Episcopal priest who died of AIDS. The mass was said by the bishop of the Archdiocese of New York, Episcopal Division, Bishop Moore. And he was in Europe; he flew back to say this mass. So the day was, ah, fairly depressing.

I can understand why. Do you live in Manhattan?

Yes, I live on the Upper West Side.

What's your health status right now?

Well, at the moment, I'm probably diagnosed with lymphadenopathy syndrome with evidence of HTLV-III antibodies, so I'm not CDC-defined AIDS. My physical status is really okay. I have lots of joint pains, I have difficulty sleeping, and I had diarrhea for about two years. Now that I'm taking this drug I'm constipated. (Laughs.)

(Laughs.) Oh, no!

I don't know if that's a side effect or not.

Do you consider that you have AIDS?

Sure, sure, I always have and I always will.

When did you first become aware of AIDS?

I became aware of AIDS somewhere around December of '81. I was aware that I was ill about four or five months before that, and in November of '81 I had a series of unexplained blackouts and eventually when I started hearing what symptoms of AIDS were, I felt that, you know, I might fit in that category.

What was the source of that knowledge of symptoms?

The Gay Men's Health Crisis was just being formed and they had posted in the bars advertising a large fundraising dance at a disco. The terms *Kaposi's sarcoma* and *GRID—Gay Related Immune Deficiency* were on the poster. Around February of '82 I was testing the hepatitis B vaccine for people who had exposure to hepatitis but didn't develop antibodies. And every time I went to that clinic, there was a little typewritten blurb about gay cancer and gay pneumonia and gay-related immune deficiency. And I started picking up that stuff and when I had read enough of it, I realized that I seemed to be falling into that category.

When was your first contact with a person with AIDS?

After I had been diagnosed in April with GRID. About June of that year I ran into severe fatigue problems which freaked me out mentally. I ended up in a support group for people with AIDS, so they were the first people that I met. After that I ran into people who had been diagnosed with AIDS or KS that I'd known previous to having joined the support group, but didn't know they had AIDS at the time.

How many people would you say that you'd had sex with before either of you were diagnosed, who now have AIDS or who died of AIDS?

Ah, two for sure, you know, people that I had contact with. One man was diagnosed with PCP after I had had sex with him, after I had been diagnosed. And one person who died; I heard through one of the hospital social workers that I was dealing with. I had had sex with him before I had the blackout experiences, and he died of KS.

How many people now do you know who have AIDS?

I would imagine about nine hundred.

How many of those people are you very emotionally close to?

Well, that's a difficult question, Lonnie. I think that, ah, I am absolutely affected by everyone who is diagnosed and everyone who dies. I would say that I have spoken to somewhere near around nine hundred people with AIDS, because for the last two years that's all I've done. And that's here in the United States and in Canada and in England.

I am very close to maybe about thirty people, very intimately, through a support group, a political person-with-AIDS committee. GMHC has a person-with-AIDS advisory committee, and I am very close with all of those people. And there are about—there are not that many people with AIDS who actually are active volunteers in GMHC, but there are three of them in the office who are very dear to me, one who just came down with PCP, and that's blown my whole month.

You know, he had lymphadenopathy for three years and then, all of a sudden, one day, not expecting it, came down with PCP. And that just frightened the hell out of me. It dropped the whole bottom out of my existence, because right now I'm feeling, "I could be next."

What was his health like just before this?

His health was very good. He was extremely cautious—he wouldn't even use the telephone without wiping it off with an alcoholic swab! He hadn't had sex in two years, he didn't drink, he didn't do drugs.

How bad were his lymph nodes?

He had lymphadenopathy, but they weren't extreme. Nothing larger than an inch. So it was really very frightening for me. Plus at the same time, another volunteer that I'm very close with had three lumps removed from his breast, so most of his breast was removed, and because there's a hospital strike going on here, they have not been able to biopsy them to let him know whether they were cancerous or not. And so he's fairly freaked out, and a third volunteer came down with KS who had not previously been sick at all, and a buddy who was a bisexual man just totally freaked out, and within one period of a week, with the clinical director who had retired and the new clinical director who was on vacation, I was responsible for handling these people. And the end result was, ah, they're doing okay right now, you know (laughs), and I'm a mess!

It's very difficult to see people going who you've been with intimately, you know, and I am in a prime position in the city with the most cases. I also work in a hospital; I work at Beth Israel AIDS Center as a volunteer, and whether they're IV drug users, Haitian women, men or women, straight or gay, I develop a relationship with these people, and we've lost maybe fifty people at Beth Israel and we've lost almost two hundred now at GMHC. And I have had contact with every one of them at one point, you know? Either close contact or first phone call or something like that.

What do all the risk groups have in common, in your perceptions of them?

Stress!

Hm. Would you say more about that?

Yeah, I'm real hot on this idea and I think that New York City is way behind in looking at things psychologically, but I feel that we are doing lots of observations of what a person goes through when they're diagnosed with what's potentially a terminal illness and the processes they go through and how they deal with stress and what they try to do with their life. But we're not doing enough about what led them to become immune-deficient, or susceptible to whatever the virus is that damages them permanently. If we could look more at reasons why a man is promiscuous rather than, you know, what's the end result of his having been promiscuous, or if we would look closer at what has driven a young person to become an IV drug user, or what does the Haitian community have to go through even after they've left their country, I think that we would come closer to what put them in the prodromal stage at which point the virus may have gone in and done permanent damage. Even given the fear that I have, I could be deceased now and I'm not. I see that most of the very politically active, angry people with AIDS in New York are still alive, and the people that I participated with in Denver last year at the National Gay Health Conference, ah, no matter what they had, PCP, KS, lymphadenopathy, what—they're all still alive, and, you know, sometimes I even feel that the people we are providing the most service for are dying and that may be the—part of the—problem. We have gone in and helped them rather than having them be angry and fight and have them do it on their own. I mean, we have done some absolutely wonderful service. All through the United States there's been incredible assistance for people with AIDS, and I'm not sure how many of those could have made it on their own. But I do see that the fighters, the angry ones, the positive ones, are doing better than the ones who have accepted it, who say "I have an illness, I'm going to die." A lot of them want it and a lot of them feel they deserve it and a lot of them feel that there is no hope, so they're not making it.

I see the same pattern of hopelessness.

Yeah, yeah. I see a strong pattern of predisposition which not a lot of people, especially the therapeutic community in New York, wants to hear about. I think some are predisposed psychologically; there are a lot of people who acknowledge in very intimate, subtle ways the fact that they're happy they're dying.

Yeah, "The world isn't worth living in," I've heard.

It's like, "Why should I be cured of AIDS? My existence sucked before. So why do I want to get better and go back to that?" There is a large group of men in New York running around trying to prove that they have AIDS. And not only gay men, but straight men. I'm right now counseling regularly a straight guy who has prostatitis, but he absolutely insists it's AIDS.

Why?

Ah, well, for the gay men I see doing that, they're men who don't relate and don't have anything to their credit that gives them self-esteem. Those of us who were open and vocal about having AIDS got some good things out of life. You know, recognition, television shows, lots of friends, people concerned about us. There's a very large percentage of people in New York who want that. And so whatever symptom they have, one swollen gland, they will spend their whole fortune going from doctor to doctor trying to get a doctor to prove that they have AIDS.

Doctor after doctor tells them, you know, "Everything looks normal; you don't have it." And they won't believe them. I've had people come to the office hysterical and just open my door and announce, "Nobody will tell me that I have AIDS, and I know I have it." These are people who are doing okay now, you know, but they went through that period.

Hm. I want to switch now, back to when you first noticed

your warning sign, like a lymph node swelling or herpes zoster.

The first warning sign for me was when I was being rolfed, and I knew my body fairly intimately because I had twenty-five sessons of rolfing, and somehow between the twentieth and the twenty-first session, I had pain in my body which I was aware were lymph glands. I had felt that the rolfer was crushing my lymph glands, so at that point I realized they were swollen. He was a gay man. Nobody knew much about AIDS, so it didn't mean much to him. And then, a few months later, after stopping that series, I started blacking out, and then I was really sure that there was something dramatic going on.

How long was it before you were diagnosed after this?

I wasn't officially diagnosed until April of 1982, and this was going on in October and November of 1981.

What were your symptoms in the summer of 1982?

Um, really very heavy fatigue. I spent almost four months in the house, not really moving very much. A limited amount of night sweats. I haven't had too many. Extreme joint pain, so that my arms were so weak that I could sometimes not pick up my own shoulder bag. I was working as a carpenter at the time. That's why I left, because one day I went to work and I couldn't lift my hammer, and it was all over from that point on.

Was your physical experience of the illness what you expected?

There wasn't much to expect because there wasn't any

knowledge at that time. The symptoms at that time were the primarily obvious ones: PCP, KS, fatigue, weight loss.

How did your gay friends react when you were told that you had GRID?

(Sighs.) Well, the people who loved me, I became very, very close with. As a matter of fact, one man who is my best friend listened to my whole life story. I told him every single thing that ever happened to me, and this was over a year and a half period. Just every night, no matter what I did, I went to his house and we smoked a joint and I just sat there and told him all my fears, all the horrible things I did, all the good things I did, all the embarrassing things I did. I mean, it was two ways. I listened to him also as he did the same thing. That was a very enlightening and lightening experience for me to get rid of all of that stuff that I might have been afraid to tell someone. Though I'm very, very open and I always have been my whole life. I mean, I would tell the most disgusting story on television—

(Laughs.)

But it was nice to have some ongoing place to unload my fears.

How about other people?

All of the superficial people in my life disappeared immediately, and that was to my advantage. You know the kind of people that call you up and say "Let's go for coffee," but when you were sitting in the restaurant you didn't really know why you were with them?

(Laughs.)

They've gone and they've never come back and I have never cultivated other people like that. You know, that kind of made things easier.

II

Without using the term *AIDS*, what is AIDS?

Um (pause) would you like the medical definition?

No, I want your opinion, your belief about what AIDS really is, without that word.

My opinion about AIDS is very metaphysical and it's not a one-sentence answer. I think that AIDS is the gay community's way of being recognized. A protest to being closeted. It's the way that we chose in our mass consciousness to get our civil rights, and if we don't get our civil rights out of this AIDS crisis, the whole thing will be, of course, futile. AIDS to the gay community is what burning buildings was to the blacks or being political is to women. It's our way of saying, "Here we are," you know, "take notice of us." I think that politics and burning buildings didn't really get people as far as they wanted. The illness is the way we chose it. We now get compassion, understanding, and helpfulness. We get people to see that there is something different about us, thrown onto us by society.

Why do some get AIDS and others do not?

It's a selection process. In that time when all of us are part of universal mind, we choose who gets what. Some people, community heroes, choose to die. Some people like me choose to get sick so that I understand the whole process, but, you know, clearly don't have any intention of dying. Some people select to be full-time volunteers. Some people select to ignore it. Some people select to fight against it, like the Moral Majority. So that is something that happens in the unconscious, or mass conscious, collective conscious, or universal mind.

What do you see the key problems for a person with AIDS to be?

Accepting the illness, being taken care of, being able to develop hope, ah (sighs), realizing that this is the time to experience quality of living, knowing that they don't have much time to go. The problem is communicating all the things that didn't work for you prior to getting this. And then, concretely, the major problems are housing and social isolation.

Is it difficult for a person with AIDS to understand how they might have unconsciously willed it to happen?

I normally don't address that subject with a person with AIDS. Mostly, people say, "It should have been me, I fucked eight thousand men in the last year!" Or they're in the other, opposite extreme, "Why me? I didn't do anything that anyone else didn't." The therapeutic community will understand what I say even though they don't know what to do with it.

Right. (Laughs.)

But the patients don't always get it. Sometimes I share my thoughts with other patients, and they'll get it, but they can't seem to do anything with it. They can't repeat it or whatnot. To them it's just like in a moment of despair it can remind them that there was some purpose. And I think one of the problems with people with AIDS or the gay community in general is that it doesn't really have a firm grasp on purpose. They're making money or going dancing or fucking or taking drugs. This crisis has put purpose back into a lot of people's lives, especially people who died and people who are serving people who are dying.

How do you perceive people are at risk for coming down with AIDS?

Exposing themselves to illness, especially if they're vulnerable. That's why I feel that some people can go to the baths constantly and not get AIDS and some people can't. My feeling is they're predisposed, so what puts them at risk is exchanging blood.

So you do think there's a virus?

I think there's a virus that does the final job, that makes it irreversible. I think there is a condition where you're susceptible to the virus that *is* reversible. I wrote a paper called "Stress: The Prodrome to Immune Deficiency," and I feel that once you're immune deficient, you may get all of that other stuff out there. My feeling still is HTLV-III or LAV is another opportunistic infection. Another one of those little things that got in there because you couldn't fend it off.

What do you think risky sex is?

Risky sex is exchanging semen, either orally or rectally. Risky sex for any illness is rimming. That's really about it.

Uh-hm. What is safe?

Um, I feel that kissing is safe, and I do kiss my lover (laughs) quite passionately. I feel that armpits are safe, nipples are safe; all the rest of the body, backs and necks. To me, my sex life looks—if you saw my lover and me in bed, it would look perfectly normal, but there are things that we will not do. Like, ah, he fucks me a lot when we're together. We're not together that often, and I have never taken his semen. We always use a condom. For the first six months we had sex, we would blow each other with a condom until I realized that I was getting blown very little because he couldn't stand the taste of the rubber!

(Laughs.)

And so eventually we lightened up on that. He has a lot of pre-come and I always wait until he's exhausted it, because usually about five minutes into foreplay it stops. Then, before I'll fuck him, he'll wash it off.

Are there any other ways that you control for catching AIDS or another infection?

I don't have sex with anyone other than Harvey, and we made the choice when we realized that we were attracted to each other that we would have sex and we would be monogamous. As far as daily living is concerned, I have been around every infectious illness that you can possibly imagine, many, many, many, many times because I work in a hospital and I don't take a lot of precautions unless the patient I'm seeing is freaked out, then I'll do it for his sake only. I have washed basins and I have washed clothes with shit in them and I have cleaned men with crypto, and I've been with people with TB and pneumocystis repeatedly. To tell you the truth, the precaution that I take is serving the community in need. My real belief is that God takes care of those who take care of others, and as long as I take care of others, my health will remain pretty stable.

Well, it has for quite a few years.

Yup. Yup. My mind is not quite as stable as my body right now, but the interesting thing is that I give blood everywhere in New York regularly to anybody that's got a study, because I feel the more I know about what's going on with me, the safer I feel. My T-cell ratio has been .3 for the last year and a half, though it had at one point gotten up to 1.25 and then dropped back down and stayed down, and my helper cells, which, in order to be in this study that I'm in they've got to be less than 600, and they've always been less than 300, and the last blood test I had before starting this experimental drug, they jumped up to 566.

Some of my glands seem smaller, though I don't really dare to check them any more. And so I almost feel like, ah, regardless of whether I'm taking this drug or not, I seem to be improving.

The whole problem with the illness is that one never knows; there is no control. Tomorrow I could either be hit by a bus or come down with PCP or get my first lesion. Even if someone came and told me that I was misdiagnosed, I would, for the next ten or fifteen years, anticipate that it might blow up in my face. I work very hard in therapy to get away from that, and even if I totally divorced myself from work around AIDS and took a regular job and moved away from New York and all of that, I will always be in fear until I'm eighty years old.

Yeah, I can see why. How do you think the government should prevent AIDS from spreading?

I don't think that the government has any control over it. Some of the things that I would like to see are money into absolutely every kind of research, the passage of universal civil rights so that people could get out of the prodromal state, and working very diligently to create a vaccine to this particular virus that they think is causing it. I *don't* want to see government intervention into stopping places that gay people can have sex! Although I would like to see all of those places eliminated, I don't necessarily want to see the government do that.

How has the AIDS crisis made you feel?

It's two and a half years now, so I can tell you that I've felt absolutely any way that you could imagine a person feeling. The day that I was diagnosed, my first reaction was, "Good, now I don't have to commit suicide." And then it went to anger that the medical profession, which was supposed to be able to cure everything, had no answers. Then it went to "I will cure myself by using vitamins and acupuncture and things like that." Now it's gone to "I'm going to be next." It's given me an incredible fear of dying. It's given me absolutely the most purpose I've ever had in my life. It's given me a reason for living. It's given me the opportunity to contribute to more people than I had ever thought possible. It's made me a media star. It's given me the exposure to educate people about what it's like to be gay, what it's like to serve and volunteer, what it's like to work with someone you morally don't believe in, and it's given me an opportunity to get over my racism and my own personal prejudices against everything, including Spanish, women, musclemen, and IV drug users. Working with all of these populations, I've had to reevaluate how I think about other people.

How do you feel about the changes in your own gay identity?

Well, I'm absolutely comfortable with who I am ninety percent of the time, and the rest of the time I'm a basket case.

(Laughs.)

You know, there are times when I feel that I don't fit, like the people that I work with. Though we try to get away from its being an elitist organization, most of the people at the Gay Men's Health Crisis have money and they go to Fire Island on the weekends. They have great clothes and private practices and stuff like that, so there are times when I realize that I'm not one of them. They know that I don't have any money at all, so they don't invite me to stay with them for the weekend on Fire Island. It's almost August and I don't have a tan; everybody else is brown. Resentment comes up, and I feel inferior or not included. Some days I have the realization that that's my victimization of myself, and it's okay to be doing what I'm doing and not being on Fire Island.

What have you felt about society's reactions to AIDS?

It's probably appropriate for what they were given to work with. Society as a whole is still in confusion and some fear, though I don't feel a lot of it because people really appreciate what they've seen me do on TV or what they've heard me say—you know, gay people and straight people. I get a lot of people who will stop me on the subway and say, "I recognize you. How do you feel?" and I know that they're interested in me. The part of society that I'm having difficulty with is the medical profession. Since 1979, they have had experience with this illness and are still overreacting. Not those people who work in AIDS clinics, but those people in the hospital network around AIDS patients. The lower education, the lower echelon you are, in the hospital, the absolute worse the treatment and the fear is. And that exists in some of the best hospitals of New York.

What emotions have you felt about people that you loved who have had AIDS?

Ah (pause), that also, I guess, spans them all. For some reason, I feel, you know, an overwhelming empathy for anyone who's ill, or anyone who dies, it doesn't even have to be from AIDS. When I hear about murder on television I get angry because there's no reason to snuff out an eleven-year-old girl's life, you know, when so many people are just dying naturally. I have a lot of anger toward people with AIDS who won't deal with their illness, though I also am understanding of that. I don't demonstrate my anger to them; I carry it around with me. I am disappointed in some people with AIDS, I am enlightened by others, I am inspired by others.

Now, if you could just give me one word that would describe your feelings about AIDS, what would it be?

(Pause.) Huh. I'm tempted to say "fear." And (pause) I'm also tempted to say "joy." You know, there's a consideration that that won't be interpreted correctly.

How do you mean it to be interpreted?

Some men who are dying are so inspiring that the feeling that I'm left with is joy mixed with pain. I've gotten so intimate with some people, you know, in the days before they left us, that, ah, the communication was so high that joy was the only thing that was left.

Those are pretty powerful experiences.

III

I want to ask you about four or five questions now about the course of the illness that you've experienced yourself. Do

you remember a time when you became ill with a cold or some other seemingly common illness before you had any sign of AIDS or GRID?

Yes. I went through a three-year period prior to blacking out, which was November of '81, in which every time I looked at a man, I came down with gonorrhea! I had three distinct, separate cases of hepatitis B and one of hepatitis A, and, unfortunately, I never had a great deal of money to play around with and I didn't trust the doctors I went to because whenever I was sick, their advice was go home and stay in bed until it's over. I didn't realize that prescription was typical of hepatitis and those kinds of viral infections. So every time I got an infection, I went to a different doctor or a different clinic, and would say to them, "What is wrong with me? You know, why do I have sex and come down with clap?" You know, I had it eight times in one year and I had sex eight times in one year! Because none of them had any record on me, they didn't see the pattern. They would just say, "It's the people you're having sex with," or "It's your dirty little life-style," or "Typical of a New Yorker," or "You faggots are all alike." Any one of a variety of statements. I knew that there was something wrong, and when I blacked out that was obvious. When I blacked out the first time I thought—and I blacked out like three times within a five- or seven-minute period—I felt that my life was over right then and there.

So that was the warning, the dramatic symptom?

Right. Right. That was the thing that told me, "Don't drink. Don't have drugs. Don't have sex anymore." I mean, all of that came long before those were recommendations. You know, while I was sitting on the floor in a bar, blacking out, thinking I was never going to wake up, that was the thought that I had: This is the time for me to stop everything.

During the time right after you found out that you had GRID, did you feel like the doctors were correct, did you accept their diagnosis?

Yeah.

What images did the diagnosis call forth?

Well, one of the things that I had heard was that Kaposi's didn't hurt. So, I was told the first day that at worst I had six to eighteen months to live. I was a carpenter at the time. I figured that every day I would go to work, and one day I wouldn't wake up. And there would be no pain.

Right after you were diagnosed, what feelings did you experience?

Um, I was happy. I didn't like the fact that I couldn't keep a relationship. At one point I got that this lifetime was to be about no relationship, and so I was so complete with that, I was happy that the life was going to be over shortly. And, as I said, you know, my first thought was, "Now I don't have to commit suicide to get out of this." I really didn't believe that I would be out of physical realities if I committed suicide.

What kinds of changes in your financial or social life occurred after that?

My whole life was about finding a lover who would stay with me the rest of my life; AIDS took that away, because immediately I thought, "Nobody wants a lover who's going to die, and now everybody is a nonpotential." AIDS took the sexual charge out of men, which was good for me. Financially, I was a carpenter and I was working free-lance. I was just about making it day to day. I had to work every day in order to eat, and once I got to the point where I couldn't work, I had to go on welfare, and it's been two years of living like a student.

After some time passed since your diagnosis, did you take stock or reevaluate your life?

The work I do represents how I've done that. I feel that I want to make a contribution. One of the disappointing things when I was diagnosed and had to quit working was that I was building these two apartments and, to me, ah, not finishing them—well, they were the only thing that I could leave, you know, to the universe. Most of the jobs that I left went out of business, so they didn't exist to begin with, and I wasn't a painter and I wasn't a writer, and so this was going to be my little legacy, and I never got to finish that. Now I guess the most important thing is that there are thousands and thousands of people who know who I am. I've either talked to them directly or they've heard me at conferences and presentations and stuff like that.

Did you ever feel like you were singled out for misfortune?

No.

You never felt like you deserved it?

I deserved it inasmuch as I didn't care to be around anymore and if there was an easy way out, you know, I, you know, um, not that I deserved it; I probably asked for it.

That's the way you sort of made sense out of the illness?

Uh-huh. I mean, I've never said, "Why me?" I've always known why me.

How have your views about life and death changed?

Well, from probably the age of fifteen to the age of thirty-nine I did not really care about being here. I always had a very strong spiritual component, not religious, but spiritual component to my life, where I didn't feel that the part of me that does feel is physical. I was always unhappy being a physical being. I didn't like my body, I didn't like my face, I didn't relate well to my surroundings. I had poor eyesight; I was always falling over everything. And I remember when I took the est training, one of the conflicts that I had with the trainer was, "How am I going to learn all the lessons possible so that I don't have to become a physical being again? I don't want to be physical." Now my feelilng is, if I die tomorrow, I think I've earned enough credits that the next trip will be easier, and I would absolutely love to live to the age of eighty, because there are so many wonderful physical things that I can enjoy and contribute to that I was not interested in for the first thirty-nine years. So it's given me the ability to enjoy walking on cement and looking at burned-down buildings and helping people.

Have your needs for emotional intimacy changed in your relationships with men?

(Sighs.) Yeah. They're not as pressing, and I have them. I have a lover. Our emotional intimacy, maybe seventy percent of it, is on the phone. I don't really get horny now, but sometimes lately I do. I used to always get horny, always be lacking physical touch. Now I get an incredible amount of hugging and kissing from friends and people that I work with. I don't have that overwhelming need to stick my cock up somebody's ass. I can be with a person and be intimate without its being sexual, and that was impossible before.

Have your beliefs about gay freedom changed any?

Yes. I feel that I am an entirely free human being, being gay. I've been gay everywhere, you know, in public. I don't mean in the gay community, I mean everywhere. I've been accepted; I've been appreciated; I've been *somewhat* understood. People empathize with me; people feel that I give them something that changed the way they thought, and I am totally aware by reading the gay press and hearing the news that the whole gay community is not in the condition that I'm in. That makes me unhappy.

How has your biological family reacted to this?

I have not heard from my brother and two sisters in two and a half years, and there was a time when I had to ask my mother not to call me any longer because she was not really supportive of me when I felt the sickest. We have a relationship again. I am actually her favorite child, though she used my being gay against me, and so does my family.

Ah, so primarily, aside from my mother, they don't exist for me. I don't have any anger any longer, although I carried it around for a good year and a half, and they are people who are not there when I need them, so, you know, biological or not, if my brother died in California I would not make an effort to go to the funeral because he wasn't there for me when I was ill, so I don't feel close to them. They have not been supportive for most of my life. I have a brother and two sisters, and once or twice a year I would call them, and once or twice a year I'd get a Christmas card or a birthday card or something, but we were not a very close family. This crisis in my life didn't contribute to making it closer.

The very interesting thing is my sister, whom I was close with through high school, was a Roman Catholic nun for eighteen years. She left the order. She now spends her life working with the terminally ill. I have had one conversation with her since I was diagnosed, during which she asked me, if I were to die, was there anything that I wanted to ask her or say to her before I did, and I thought to myself, "Wow! At last, you know, the ability to communicate."

Yeah!

And I never saw her again, and I never heard from her again, never had a card, never had a—anything. And the question that I asked her was, "Are you gay?" And I'm absolutely clear that she is. Her three roommates are the most dikey women that you've ever seen in your life, and she said no, she wasn't. You know, and then I thought, well, this level of communication just dropped to an all-time low. You lied to me and I'm dying, so it didn't matter. So—(Chuckles and sighs.)

What about other biological families? Does it seem like other people with AIDS bring their biological families in as supportive or pretty much like they've always been?

Well, I've seen just everything you could imagine. I've seen people who had a son in the hospital in New York and they lived in Florida and they moved up here and never left the hospital the whole time he was hospitalized, and became very intimate and close. And I've seen people who just totally threw their person-with-AIDS out of their home. And I have seen people who totally ignored two gay men who had a twenty-five-year relationship and the day that one died, the family drove the truck up and emptied everything out of the apartment. And I've seen parents who would take the son out of the hospital and take him to another city and not allow his two-or three-year lover to be part of the dying process or the burial or any of that.

I've seen everything. I've seen some people who are just

wonderfully, wonderfully supportive, and I've seen people who just totally threw out the gay person, like he never existed—and blamed him! I've seen people actually call Jerry Falwell and have him try to contact the person with AIDS to get him to change his sexual preference. You know, all kinds of disgusting things and all kinds of beautiful things have happened here.

What about mainstream medicine?

Um, boy, they don't know a lot! (Laughs.) You know, when I started reading about immunology and realized that I could not find a book that was written before 1968, I realized how little they know. And I think they do, too, and I think it's real hard on the medical profession. I think a lot of the anger that doctors sometimes demonstrate to their patients comes out of the futility of not being able to save people when their whole life was about that.

That would be very frustrating. What do you think would be an effective relationship between medicine and government?

(Sighs.) I don't think I know how to answer that question.

How do you think medicine does relate to government?

As big business relates to government.

What about homeopathic medicine? How does it define and treat people with AIDS differently than mainstream medicine?

Well, the only homeopathic treatment I think will have

any effect on AIDS is acupuncture, especially around the issue of fatigue. I think that acupuncture really has given people more strength. I see it in men who are on chemotherapy, who would go from their chemotherapy to their acupuncture clinic and got through that experience with very few side effects. Some people did not lose their hair, and I think that acupuncture had something to do with that.

What about macrobiotics?

Macrobiotics, I think, is a complete waste for anyone with AIDS. It's too difficult on the body, it's too major a change, and it's irritating on its own. I don't think a person with AIDS has the stamina to wait for the body to stabilize on that kind of diet.

Psychic healers—and I've been to a few myself—seem to be relatively ineffective. Though psychologically they might make the process easier, I have not seen a psychic healer save anyone. Ah (sighs), what are some others? Chiropractic doesn't do much. I am opposed to people using small doses of poisons to clean out the body. That's not effective at all, from what I've seen.

Bob, you mentioned earlier that you thought one of the reasons why people get AIDS was that it was a mental illness and something that varies with one's will to live. What's the goal, ultimately, for yourself? Is it still to die? (Pause.) Since you were diagnosed, have you changed your mind?

Yup, yup. that's a difficult thing for me to give you a great answer on. I'm not sure that the end result is going to be living to eighty. That's what I say that I want it to be.

Uh-huh. But why do you now want to live? Society isn't becoming pro-gay now. What made a difference for you?

Seeing that I was big enough to do what I've always wanted to do. We used to make key tags and I used to work ten or twelve hours a day, six days a week, and at least once every six months I thought, "If it was only people rather than key tags that I was putting this amount of effort into." And now I'm doing that. I didn't need to live to be the king of key tags. And I wouldn't mind living long enough to be the king of people. If someone were to describe me as the Kübler-Ross of the gay community, I would be real pleased. I would say that I had accomplished my goal.

I have a problem with accomplishing my goal, because I feel that death is the next thing after having accomplished your goal. I have gone through fear that once I've gotten to a point where I'm capable of accomplishing my goal, death may be the end result. I could be a two-year hero rather than a forty-year hero. And so I'm not really clear whether I have developed the right mindset to stay alive for forty years, though I at least have thoughts that I want to. Ultimately it may be that having gotten this condition, it has done irreversible damage.

Is it possible to reverse it by positive thinking?

I think that it is, yes. You know, but that's the kind of question I'd have to tell you at the age of seventy-nine.

Right! (Laughs.)

Feeling that I'm right and convincing myself that I'm right are not always the same thing. You know, sometimes there is a fear that my life was supposed to be over at forty-four and all of this contribution is just what I did up to the age of forty-four and I'm never going to go beyond that, you know, no matter how much good I do. Now the good may have results beyond this life. It may mean that I don't have to come back as a physical being again, and it may be that I could, you know, get five steps closer to heaven or whatever is out there. It may mean that I come back as a spiritual being and influence things on the planet, but I don't have to live here myself.

That wouldn't be bad, huh? (Laughs.)

Yeah, it wouldn't. I don't know if you've ever read books like the Seth material, but they are written by someone who used to be physical and dictates them through somebody who still is.

Oh, yes! I have one of those: *Seth Speaks*.

Seth Speaks, right. The books that came after that—there's two or three that are just mind-boggling. One of them is called *The Nature of Personal Reality*, and it's about six hundred pages. If you ever wanted to get into some reading about someone who tells you what life is about from the point of view of somebody who's been here and isn't any longer and can now observe the whole thing, they are incredibly enlightening. And they explain what living is, they explain what dying is, they explain what epidemics are, they explain what catastrophes are, and, you know, when I can hold that knowledge as a part of me, I am comfortable with what's happening and when I can't, I'm freaked out.

Well, it sounds to me like you've really grounded your view of yourself in what's going on around you and you've got a pretty clear image of it.

If you were working with me in the office in the last two weeks, you'd probably say, "Poor Bob has decompensated."

(Laughs.) Well, we all have our moments. How do you feel about the interview?

I feel very comfortable. It got me out of my low feelings of having gone to a funeral today.

I send you a big hug and lots of support for what you're going through right now.

Thank you.

3

A Double Whammy

Lance Gaines

Lance Gaines moved from Cleveland to San Francisco to seek medical care for Kaposi's sarcoma and full-blown (frank) AIDS.* His diagnosis at age twenty-one and his disclosure of homosexuality to his parents coincided. A junior corporate auditor for the IRS, this young man experienced the anguish of AIDS amid the whirlwinds of coming out.

When did you first learn about AIDS?

I never heard about it until I saw a special on it on "20/20." That was about seven months before I was diagnosed.

Was this television special the only place that you heard about it, or did you hear about it from other sources?

That was the first time I heard about it. The local newspapers started printing the AP wires from San Francisco about seven months after that, when I was diagnosed.

Did you see lesions before diagnosis? How long ago were you aware something was going on with your body?

---

*The San Francisco service agency that referred Lance Gaines to be interviewed later notified me that he had left San Francisco before confirming his diagnosis.

Well, I knew something was going on. I got diagnosed in September of '83. I knew something was going wrong around July, but I figured if I gave myself a little bit of time I would be okay, you know. I figured maybe I had a flu virus or something like that, but toward August I started to feel really shitty and noticed the lesions and had a flashback on that thing I saw on "20/20." The special I saw had a man with lesions in it. Mine looked kind of like that, so I went to one of the clinics and they referred me to my own doctor. I went to my doctor, and he told me I had AIDS.

Did you know anyone else with AIDS at that time?

No, I didn't. The first time I met someone else with AIDS was about December of '83. That was back in Cleveland.

How close were you to that person?

Not very, not very close at all.

If you could describe what is happening to your body without using the word AIDS, how would you describe it?

(Long pause.) Literally, just degenerating. That's about all I can say, just deteriorating. I am losing all my strength.

Where do you think you caught this from?

To tell you the truth, it had to be from sex. That's all it could be from.

How do you perceive your risk now for becoming ill from other infections?

I feel it's pretty good. I've got to take very good care of

myself. I've got to be very careful and really watch myself, you know, like around people with colds. I've got a very severe cough and very severe cold right now. I just haven't been feeling too well.

Lance, would you tell me how many KS lesions you have?

I've got forty-three lesions on the outside of my body and I have twenty-one on the inside.

How did they know how many you have on the inside?

When I was in Cleveland, they gave me this fluid and I drank it. It went into my system and—

They did a CAT scan?

Yeah, and I have them on the inside of my lungs and going down my throat.

What day were you diagnosed?

September second of '83.

That is just about the same time I was diagnosed with KS. When did you tell your parents?

I didn't tell my parents until I couldn't put it off.

Are the lesions in visible places externally?

At first they were down around the groin area. Now they've moved up where they're quite apparent.

And are you on treatment?

I go for chemotherapy, plus I'm taking vitamins A, B, and C.

How often do you get chemotherapy?

Once a week.

You moved here because you wanted better medical care?

Yeah—quite true!

What was your health experience like in Cleveland?

The doctors were very poor. They were very anti-AIDS victim. They did not care for "those kind of people." There were only a few AIDS patients—three serious cases in Cleveland—when I was there. There are, you know, more minor cases, the gray cloud cases.

What treatment did they give you?

The treatment was very poor and full of "attitude." They wouldn't give me any answers. I've just started my chemotherapy. I haven't had my first session yet. All they treated me with there was vitamins. My doctor told me that there was nothing else they could do for me there, other than the Cleveland clinic. My doctor suggested that I move out here.

Did you have people to come to in San Francisco?

No. I know nobody in the city.

Where are you living?

I live in a Shanti* residence.

*A San Francisco–based social service agency providing counseling and support to people dealing with AIDS and other potentially life-threatening illness.

What would you consider your sexual identification?

I've always been gay. Well, since I was about fifteen or so—about six years.

What is Cleveland's gay community like?

Cleveland has a very different kind of gay community. The bathhouses there are the most dirty things you've seen in your life. They still haven't cleaned them up—even with the AIDS epidemic. They are literally filthy.

When you're around other people now with AIDS, how do you control your risk for getting something else?

Nothing—all I do is take vitamins.

What is your environment like at the Shanti residence?

There's one man here at Shanti who is going to die. He weighs sixty-seven pounds, he's so sick. We've got another man here who is forty-five years old, and he's lost his mind. He weighs about eighty pounds, and he's lost his mind. He will walk around just in a daze. We've got another man here who's given up. I tell you, it's starting to affect me, because their attitude is so poor. They don't want to live anymore; I want to live very badly, and (pause) it gets very confusing. These people have just totally given up; I've got too many things I want to do.

How have you changed physically since your diagnosis?

When I was first diagnosed, I weighed 242 pounds. I weighed 178 pounds when I went to the doctor today. I eat like a pig now, and last week I lost four and a half pounds. I'll drink milkshake after milkshake, but I just cannot stop losing. I used to be able to throw a sixteen-pound ball—no problem. I was so big! Now it's starting to get very hard to throw even a fifteen-pound ball. When I go bowling, I can bowl maybe four games, and I'm pooped. I go home, fall over, and fall asleep.

Since you were diagnosed, have you noticed any changes in your needs for intimacy?

Yeah. I've found out that I'm looking more for companionship, a lover type, more than sex.

Have your relationships with other men changed for the better?

Not quite. At first, I was afraid—I really was—I felt like a freak.

Have you felt sort of ostracized from the gay community?

Yes! In Cleveland I did. I haven't gone to one bar yet in San Francisco. I've gone to Shanti and back, from the Pride Foundation. I'm afraid to go out by myself, you know.

Is that a new feeling for you?

Yes. I've kind of been to myself, which is not like me. I'm very wild; I mean, you know, like a free spirit, taking things as they come. I used to like going out and running around all night long, and things like that.

Have you gone out with anyone to party or meet people here yet?

Well, the other night I went to an AA meeting, because of

someone who was alcoholic who works there. He asked me to come along. He introduced me to his friends. I was walking back by Post and Polk, when I walked past some guy lying on the ground. He was crying, and he was very badly beaten up. When I looked down, I saw that it was somebody from the AA meeting who had AIDS.

Well, what had happened?

Uh, his lover had beaten him up. Remember the article in the *Examiner?* The one that explained where the AIDS patients were living and all of that?

Yes!

I was one of "them" living there.

The hotel Mayor Feinstein removed every one of "those people" from?

That's right.

Where did the others go?

I can't say, but I know where they all are now, and I knew where they all were then. Anyway, it was one of the people whom I had met, who had lived there; his lover was the person who had called the *Examiner*. His lover was the one who has serious KS. I will state a first name. It was John who had serious KS. He was the one who called the *Examiner*. Tommy had just gotten diagnosed, and his lover had beaten him up and—thank God they were staying in different hotel rooms, even if it was in the same place. And so I picked up Tommy, and I was sick, but I carried him, literally, two blocks before we could get a taxi. They were running all over, empty ones. I

could not get one! It took me two blocks before I could get one.
Then Tommy was so scared to tell anybody where he was staying, even me, that it took me about a half hour and $21 taxi
fare before I could get out of him where he lived! I finally got
him home and calmed him down to where he could talk. He is
so afraid of the gay community, because he has AIDS. He is
actually thinking about going back to John!

How has AIDS changed your values about life and death?

My family has a very long lifespan, and I figured, well, I
would, too. My great-grandmother lived to be 105, and just
died two years ago. My grandmother now is seventy-seven,
and in perfect health. My grandmother and my grandfather,
my mother's parents, are alive. My father's parents are alive
and everybody's doing well. Very long lifespans, and I figured,
I'm going to live a good, long time. Life was quantity, but now
it's quality. I mean, for the first time in my life, I want to do
things for other people. It makes me feel better now, to do
things for other people. Do you know what I mean?

Yeah. What about death? What do you think happens?

I don't know. I'm—I'm—I'll be truthful about it. I'm quite
frightened about it, I really am. I really don't understand it. I'm
kind of afraid of it, but when it comes, it comes. But at least I'll
have the satisfaction of what I've done with stuff, you know?

Yes, I do know.

I mean, I've done as much as I can.

Yes. Your spirit is noble, and no one can take that.

That's right, and I'll know that I've at least tried to accom-
plish something, tried to help in every way I could.

You mentioned earlier some things about your biological family. Is there anything that you want to add about them?

My family has responded very poorly. They treat me like a black sheep. Most families that I know and most families that are straight and up-to-date, who know what's going on by only seeing me on the street, stare at me.

Uh-huh. Do you think that's because the KS lesions are so obvious?

Yeah.

How about organized medicine? What's your impression about the way they've dealt with it?

That all depends. In Cleveland it was very poor. You can't even call it *organized* medicine. You can just call it medicine. Out here I've been treated better. I've been treated much better. But the thing is, it's so crowded here! I went yesterday to the hospital to get some Demerol. I walked past Ward 86 and they've got fourteen new AIDS patients that were diagnosed *this* week!

How effective do you think alternative medicine is in treating AIDS?

The vitamins haven't done a damn thing for me. They really haven't. All they do is make me tired. That's about it. They've got all kinds of stuff here. Hypnotists and all that.

Yeah, everything. But, buyer beware! Did you have any reactions from organized religion before you left Ohio?

I'm not welcome in my Catholic church anymore. I was politely asked not to return to the church by the monsignor.

What's your perception of how the media have dealt with this?

Well, the straight media has been a pain in the ass, they really have: They're hounding everybody, even down at the AIDS Foundation, they're hounding everybody. They hound, and they're pushy. I think the TV handles it well. They can be rude at times, and stuff, but I think they do quite well. But the thing I'm most disappointed with is the gay media. Like in the *B.A.R.*, the *Sentinel*, all of them. I think the *B.A.R.* [*Bay Area Reporter*] is the worst, because all you see when you open it up, all you see on every one of those pages, is the word AIDS. It's okay to be informed, but you don't want to cause a panic. I don't know what they're gonna do if they keep that up, because I have AIDS and I get sick of opening up the front page and seeing the word AIDS enlarged; and you turn the page, and it's AIDS, AIDS, AIDS everywhere. I think on one or two pages is fine, but not the whole thing. I may have AIDS, yeah, but there's more to life than AIDS.

How is the AIDS epidemic going to change the way our society treats homosexuality?

I think they're gonna look down on it even more than they do now.

What do you think the gay movement's agenda will be for the future?

I really think the gay movement and sexual liberation are going to slow down for a while, until there is a breakthrough with AIDS. Gays just can't have sex a lot during the AIDS scare. If there's going to be any kind of gay movement during the AIDS epidemic, it's going to have to be on individual rights.

Individual choice and self-determination is what the movement was supposed to be about all along.

Yeah. I don't think it can be on the idea that we should be able to have sex with this and that person, just because we want to. It's going to have to be individual. It's going to have to be like civil rights for humans. You're going to have to include lesbians, too. You know, it can't just be a gay men's movement. It will have to be a gay and lesbian movement.

Yeah, I agree! In terms of coming out, how has AIDS changed the whole coming-out process? You ought to be able to speak to this, because it happened right at the same time for you.

(Laughs.) It was very, very rough. My family really did make me look at myself again. I didn't have the self-confidence that I do now. I should have been more stable. I shouldn't have had to say, "Well, you're a bad person." I shouldn't have had to go through that. But now I can honestly say that I know I'm not a bad person. It was very hard for me to come out when I had AIDS, because it was like a double whammy for everybody that I knew.

Have you changed since your diagnosis?

Yeah, I think I have. If you could see how much I've changed since I got diagnosed! I was very snotty, very hoity-toity, Mr. Wonderful. Now I've realized that I'm just one in twenty billion, or however many there are on this earth. I am special in my own way, but there are people better than me. I came to realize that I'm not God's gift to the gay community like I thought I was.

I think the more we see this as a shared thing, the less we

blame ourselves. We're able to bond together and make something else out of it. We can make it a real move toward humanity, instead of persecuting individuals for their assumed filthiness.

I think we're going to see less people coming out now. I really do.

I think that we will, too. If the truth were told about the human experience, we would see fewer people coming out like the stereotypical "gay," and more people having sexual ethics. People could be more human with each other and less categorical. I hope this is what happens. This is my vision of a better world. What's your vision of a better world?

For me, it would be that there wouldn't even have to be a "thing" called *gay*. There shouldn't even have to be a "thing" called *straight*. Everybody should just be able to do their own thing. Nobody should be allowed to interfere. I told my father, I said, "Why should it make any difference to you if I want to go to bed and fuck a mouse? Because it's my business, not yours, and if I do what belongs to my business, it doesn't make me any less of a man. It doesn't make a woman any less of a woman if she wants to go to bed with another woman. As a matter of fact, it makes me more of a man than you, because I'm willing to admit what I am and what I want to do. I have feelings, and it makes me more of a man. I'm not afraid to cry, and I've never seen you cry once."

4

My Roommate Breaks Dishes

Jeff

Jeff is a twenty-nine-year-old gay man with AIDS. He was diagnosed with Pneumocystis carinii pneumonia (PCP). Living in Salt Lake City, Jeff is an example of the widespread pattern of AIDS in America: He has fought as an AIDS activist in Utah.

When did you first become aware of AIDS?

About a year and a half ago.

Where did you learn about it? Was it through the media, friends?

Through the media and then getting hit with it in Omaha.

What do you mean?

That's where I was diagnosed.

Oh. What was your first contact with a person with AIDS?

This other guy in Omaha had it. He died from it. We became kind of good friends.

How many people do you know right now who have AIDS?

I know of about five others. I know me, and somebody else that they're not sure about.

How close are you to these other people?

The one that they're not sure about, I'm real close to. The other people, I'm not real close to.

Do they live close to you?

I don't really know. We're trying to start a support group.

Your physical distance is close enough that you could do that?

Yeah.

Okay. What stages of illness are these other people in?

One has KS. One that I know of just got out of the hospital from having PCP.

When did you first notice some kind of warning sign, like a lymph node swelling or herpes zoster or something like that?

About a year and a half ago, I noticed I started getting real lumpy in my lymph nodes, and they didn't go away. I was in a little town of 10,000 people and they put me in the hospital there. While I was there, I lost a whole bunch of weight and started having diarrhea. They couldn't figure out what was wrong with me. I had a choice of getting transferred to Omaha, Nebraska, or Des Moines, Iowa, and I went to Omaha because that's where my family's at.

What was the date of your diagnosis?

Two days after Easter.

And when you were diagnosed, what symptoms did you present with?

All the general ones: lymphadenopathy, night sweats, diarrhea, thrush, and at the time I had PCP.

Was your physical experience of the illness what you expected?

I didn't expect that it would hit so hard. It's real scary being in a protective isolation room for so long.

Was your perception of the ways that others reacted to you what you expected?

No, I felt like a leper. I had one good nurse, who was always bright and cheerful.

If you could describe what's happening with your body without using the term *AIDS*, how would you define what AIDS is?

It's when your body's immune system forgets to hand you its resignation and goes on a vacation for the rest of its days.

(Laughs.)

I've learned through all this I have to maintain my sense of humor.

Well, congratulations, you have! (They both laugh.) How do you believe AIDS is spread?

I feel that it's a virus. They're real close to finding what virus it is, so they can give people a cure if they catch them in time.

What would you say are the key problems for a person with AIDS?

Adequate health-care coverage, either through Medicare or Medicaid or a combination of both. Also, adequate or low-rent housing. A support network that would have a toll-free number (like the National Gay Task Force has). PWAs need to have a support group that's always there just to talk to people with AIDS. It should be open twenty-four hours a day.

Do you have those things?

No. We've got people on the social services here that are on our side, who are pushing for us to get state-given medical cards so we can get free health care.

Is making the decision between mainstream treatments and alternative treatments something that is a key problem? Are you able to make a good decision about your treatment?

It's hard to make a good decision, because you really don't know. We're like stuck here. The only thing they can do is treat the symptomatic, opportunistic infections when they come up. They really don't know what to do.

Are you on any treatments now?

Not really. Just going to the doctor and getting antibiotics once in a while to treat some infection.

What made you at risk for catching AIDS?

They're not real sure how I got it. They think that I'm one

of the people that got it in a blood transfusion. But I'm going, "Well, everybody's at risk," you know, if it's supposed to be that way.

How do you think other people with AIDS are at risk for catching other infections?

Well, if they do things so they're not in the high risk for catching other infections, they shouldn't have anything to worry about. You know, if they keep protecting themselves. One of my big things, and I'm not doing it right, is, if you have cats, to use rubber gloves when you change their cat box. We didn't have any rubber gloves around the house, so I figured, well, bare hands and lots of soap and water and I ought to be okay. But they're not real sure. I just think that if you're keeping yourself halfway healthy, as hard as it is to try to do that, and just do what the doctors tell you, you shouldn't have any problems. If you think you're getting something, get to the doctor real quick.

Right! What about sex? What do you think is risky sex?

Fist fucking, I guess. Also water sports.

What is safe?

Is anything safe?

(Laughs.) Do you believe these definitions, this "risky" versus "safe" sex stuff? What do you think about that?

If I pick up somebody and go to bed with them, I make sure I don't come in them or vice versa. I figure the chances of somebody contracting it from me, personally, is like one in a million.

Why?

I feel that whatever it is that originally makes you sick,

that weakens your immune system, is a caustic agent that has already done its damage and is already out of your body. It'd be like a tick sucking on you for a while and then leaving and finding somebody else. They've spread what little diseases they're going to spread to you. It's kind of hard to maintain a "Should I be celibate or not?" attitude when you know as well as I do that sex is fun.

(Laughs.) How do you think the government should intervene and stop AIDS from spreading?

I think that they should give more funding to research places so a causative agent and/or treatments and/or cure could be found. They need to quit spending so much overseas and start cycling some of it here.

I'm going to switch now to your emotional reactions to AIDS.

Okay.

How has the AIDS crisis made you feel?

At first, I felt real hurt, real upset. I thought, "What did I do to deserve this?" After I started thinking about it real logically, which took a while, and started listening to people who kind of knew what they were talking about when it first hit, I kind of got over it.

What kinds of emotions have you experienced in response to your own well-being and AIDS?

I'm real cautious. If I even start to feel the least little bit sick, I make the quickest appointment to the doctor I can get. It's hell knowing that you might not be around tomorrow.

But you would like to be around tomorrow?

Oh, boy, would I ever! I'd like to be around till I'm eighty or ninety. I'd like to be one of the old trolls that sit in a bar and look at all the pretty young men walk in! And just sit back and remember.

Did you feel that way before you were diagnosed?

Yeah.

What kinds of changes have you experienced in terms of your gay identity?

I've, like, found out who my friends are. I found out that not all families come running together when a crisis like this hits. That another family member can't quite deal with it, and it takes a while before they come around to it. I've been barred from bars because people are afraid of the fear that I spread because I have AIDS. And I'm going, "Look, guys, I've got hard-core, in-writing stuff that says I'm not a health hazard or anything else."

How does it make you feel, when they react like that?

It makes me feel like a leper at times. And then I just figure, "Okay, well, if you want to be idiots and be part of the general panic, then go right ahead, be my guest, but I'll still stand here and have my literature to back me up." I'm kind of trying to be an AIDS activist again. In Omaha, after it was diagnosed and confirmed, I came flying out of the closet totally. TV, radio, newspaper, making the public aware, having information available. Because of my coming out of the closet, Omaha got mobile testing stations off the drawing board and into the streets.

What was your hope in doing that? What was your intention?

That if I can help to early diagnose another fellow family member, since we are all one big family, then so be it. I'm starting to get those feelings for Salt Lake.

If you could summarize your reaction to AIDS, what one word best describes your feelings about AIDS?

There's not really one word I could use, but two: anger and hurt.

Do you remember a time when you became ill with a cold or some seemingly common illness before you had any sign of AIDS? Were you especially sensitive to some kinds of physical illnesses?

Right before diagnosis, I had a cold that hung on for like a month and a half.

What else was going on with you right then?

I was just real weak. I'm just, like, hangin' out now, you know?

Uh-huh. Do you remember a time when you became ill with something that really alarmed you, and what sent you to the doctor? Something you really thought might mean that you had AIDS? What was it that brought you to present yourself to the doctor?

The fevers.

That was the warning cue?

Yeah, I started running a fever all the time. And I went to the doctor and they couldn't figure out what it was, so they put me in the hospital.

When they told you that you had AIDS, did you believe them?

I told them I wanted a second opinion.

What images came to your mind when they told you you had AIDS?

That within six months I'd be sitting in a wheelchair and my face would be swollen real grossly. I'd be on oxygen and gasping for breath and eventually, ah, kick off.

What did that make you feel?

Real uncomfortable. Real upset. Real sick. Just being told the diagnosis and the stigma of it—for a while—will make you feel sicker than you might really be. You're sick, but then all of a sudden they tell you you have AIDS and you feel just like all the hope and all the strength that you've been trying to build up just gets zapped out from underneath you.

What happened in terms of your economic and social life?

Let's see, my social life was drastically cut back. At that point I found out who my friends were. I had a gay couple— well, there were two gay couples, one a lesbian who would come up to the hospital every day and see me, and the other couple would come up on weekends. (Sneezes.) Excuse me. I think my allergies are acting up. I'm allergic to something that's in the air.

Right after you were diagnosed, like maybe a week after

or something like that, after the initial shock of the diagnosis, did you feel like you had been singled out for misfortune?

I did, but at the same time, I also felt that I got singled out to be a test.

What do you mean?

Like, the person upstairs was making me a guinea pig.

Did you reevaluate your life?

Oh, yeah, a number of times.

What parts of your life did you think about?

My ability to have a lover again.

Do you have a lover now?

No. I've got a roommate. They're not real sure of the diagnosis yet. They're saying it could be AIDS, but they're not sure.

Why did you wonder whether or not you could have another lover?

I just have. I don't really want to be alone, and I've got my roommate and we're real close, but yet I like the familiarity of having the same person wake up next to you in the morning and just give you a hug and a kiss and say "Good morning." And have somebody tell you that they love you, you know, come up and put their arms around you and just tell you that they love you.

Did you feel that no one would want to be your lover?

Yeah, after what happened in the hospital.

What happened?

When I found out I had AIDS, I turned to my lover real
quick, even before I told my folks, and it backed him up. There
were 120 miles between us and I could hear his voice over the
phone get real funny, and he quit coming down to see me. I
got out of the hospital and went back to Creston, and at first
he was real happy to see me home. It's like, "It didn't kill him.
He's home. Maybe he's okay." And then things just kind of
got worse between us. Finally, I started getting sick again and I
had to get back to Omaha, and since my family lives in Omaha
I figured, well, live there.

**During that time when he was distancing himself from
you, how did you make sense out of your illness? What did it
mean to you?**

It meant that I just lost someone very dear whom I loved,
and I didn't like that. It made me—it made me feel like a real
sleazebag.

**When you were evaluating yourself, what else did you
think about?**

There were things that I definitely couldn't do anymore,
and it hurt to give up old party favorites. There are places that
I used to like to go party that I can't go to anymore.

**One of the great things about having AIDS is that now
people take me seriously and they don't treat me like just
pretty party man.**

Uh-huh. That's the one nice thing I've found out about it,
too.

How have you changed since you became aware that you had AIDS?

That's really difficult to put my finger on. Let's see. I'm more of a homebody.

How has your view of yourself as a gay man changed?

It's difficult to say. I went through some real heavy-duty emotional problems because of this. I think I got that all straightened out. I still think I'm a reasonably good-looking gay guy.

How have your values about life and death changed?

I'm more inclined to want to live, but I've reconciled myself to the fact that when it comes that time, that everything will be okay, too.

If you could live as many years as you would like to, how many would you say you'd like to live?

Ah, probably till I'm eighty. Fifty years, maybe.

Since you were told that you might die pretty soon, has your concept of time changed? I mean, do your days seem longer or shorter?

The days seem longer; the nights seem real short.

Is there anything about the experience that you think that you would really like for people who might read this to know about what it feels like to have AIDS?

Oh, boy, live each minute to the max, because we don't

get another chance! If somebody who reads this hasn't had it and kind of wants to know what it feels like, I think it feels like having a real bad case of the flu where you're not sure if you have to puke or poop and not sure which end to put over the toilet first. When that's over, you're just so drained. That's what you feel like when you wake up in the morning, for no reason. It's really getting to be the pits. It's different going from being a semihealthy, active gay guy to somebody who has to watch what they do all the time. It takes a lot to get used to it, and I'm still not used to it. I still have my bad days, I'm just like anybody else.

But you manage the course of the illness, whether it goes up or down?

Yeah, I have to.

What kinds of things do you do to compromise, so you can kind of stay normal in living?

Oh, I've got an answering service. I have also got call forwarding on my phone, so that if I don't want to be bothered, I'll forward it to the answering service. For some reason, all of my next-door neighbors are losing their minds and they're all running to me, so I'll forward calls to places like "Dial-an-Atheist" or "Time and Temperature" or, since we're here in Salt Lake City, home of the Mormons, I forward it to the LDS Church Office Building!

(Laughs.) You're great! So there really are great ways to cope with all of it?

Yeah, if I don't want to be disturbed, I hang my little sign out front on my door that says, "To Whom It May Concern: We're asleep. If you value your life, don't wake us up. If you wake me up, you'd best give your soul to God, because your ass will be mine."

(Laughs.)

And nobody bothers us. Or we'll forward the phone to the answering service and tell them to tell people that, yes, we're home, but that they shouldn't count on very much, because we're having a crisis or something.

It sounds like you don't believe pestilences are for pure sin.

That's right! We also get rid of the—the hurt and the anger and all the stress that goes along with having it. My roommate breaks dishes.

Oh, no!

We went through so many dishes, we're going to have to go down to Deseret and pick up plates for ten cents apiece.

(Laughs.) That's funny.

For two days, we were picking shrapnel up out of the bedroom, and the bedroom is a long way from the kitchen.

Well, whatever works.

I will get away and go down—I've got my master's degree in music—to a music store at VCMI Center, which is about two blocks away, where I know the guy that is the musician salesman there. And I sit down and play one of their organs for like two hours. I also do poetry. I'm also starting my own little parish church.

Of what religious belief?

Interdenominational. I was a Roman Catholic priest for a
while.

**Interesting! I'm a Southern Baptist minister. (They
laugh.)**

I read that. And I have a way of preaching that is normally
considered Bible-banging Southern Baptist or real heavy-duty,
Jerry Falwell type. It used to freak the Catholics out. I still
preach up a storm. I've got some real strange people in my
congregation. One guy's losing his mind; he thinks he's King
Tut!

Oh, no! Life is never dull, Jeff.

5

Just Like a Heart Attack

John

John is a thirty-six-year-old gay man with Kaposi's sarcoma, diagnosed in October 1983. He was living in Oakland at that time, and has since moved to San Francisco. He is an accountant.

When did you first learn of AIDS?

Oh, about the time that Mark Feldman was diagnosed, which was around November of '82.

Where did you get most of your information about AIDS?

From Mark.

Without using the term *AIDS*, describe what you feel happening to your body.

AIDS is something comparable to a heart attack, where I had a very serious illness. Just like a heart attack, your body can't ignore the message that it's received as far as a health threat to your life. But at the same time, by nurturance of self, you can survive and overcome the situation. That's my attitude about AIDS.

So in place of *AIDS* you use *heart attack*. You really didn't have a heart attack.

My body had a reaction, a deathlike situation like you would if you had a heart attack, and by proper treatment and care I will be able to be fine and survive. But if I don't, then the symptoms and things are going to continue to progress just like a heart attack, and you have a second heart attack which will kill you.

What would you say that the odds are that you will live another year?

(Laughs.) Boy, that's a hard question to answer. Uh, I guess fifty-fifty. I'm not sure.

What are the odds that you think you will die of a heart attack in the next year?

Not very good at all. I'm real clear that I'm pretty healthy. Probably the odds would be one to a hundred.

What do you think the odds are for becoming ill with some other opportunistic infection that will be fatal in the next year?

Fifty-fifty.

What do you think your risk is for being in a car accident in the next year?

One in a thousand.

What do you think your risk is in being killed in some kind of accident other than a car accident in the next year?

Oh, about one in a hundred.

When you are with other people who have AIDS, are you aware that you are at risk for contracting their illnesses?

I'm aware of it, yeah.

And how much do you feel that you are at risk for contracting other people's illnesses in general?

Mild. It would probably be like one in ten or something.

What are the odds that you would die of a nuclear disaster in the next year?

Fifty-fifty. Especially with Ronald Reagan's hostility. (They laugh.)

Is there anything you've noticed since your diagnosis as far as health?

I'm finding myself vulnerable to some irritating health problems like rashes and such. But I don't feel that they're life-threatening. I feel like they're a test. I do observe a lot of people around me and I'm real upset that a lot of them are simply in the process of dying. I watch people around me just get weaker and weaker and sicker and sicker and not survive.

Do you do anything around those people to control your risk for contracting illnesses from them?

I go around them and try to get them to come back alive. I mean, I'm trying to sell them on the idea of coming back to life. I don't feel the least bit threatened. I feel that part of the destruction of these people is their attitude, but I don't feel the least bit threatened by going around them as far as them damaging my attitude. And as far as health is concerned, I already have the disease. I don't really know outside of the opportunity for some other opportunistic disease to come around me. I don't feel that I'm any more at risk than I already am. I think that PCP is probably the only one that I'm really concerned with, because there's probably a real good possibility that I need to be real careful around people who are actively sick.

What about your emotional experience with AIDS? How did you feel when you found it out?

When I found out about Mark Feldman, I felt a sharp sense of loss, it really didn't seem appropriate to me to be threatened. I felt a deep sense of loss and grief, you know, about this person. I admired his braveness. But I was angry. I felt like maybe the gay community as a whole was under siege in some ways, in the respect of the AIDS phobia, the labeling. I think that it's been really a tragedy how the American press has made this into a gay disease.

I do, too.

Which means that people have a little less initiative to try to do something to cure the disease.

Yeah. We can talk about that, but right now I want to try to get to focus on the content of the emotions that you've had since you've had it.

Since I was diagnosed, I've gone through a roller coaster of feelings, and sometimes, even now, there are days when I'm very upset about it. I'm very vulnerable as far as my feelings.

Vulnerable? Do you mean other people can have an impact on your emotions more easily, or you're more sensitive to your own emotions? How do you mean?

I'm vulnerable to other people's negative attitudes about

AIDS. But I also feel very discouraged, and basically I'm not real clear how I'm going to survive or if I'm going to survive at all, or even if I want to survive.

Do you still feel that way?

Yes, I'm not really sure that I want to survive. I wish it was over.

What do you do on those days?

Just . . . carry on. Yeah, I just progress with the day.

How has AIDS influenced the whole notion of coming out as a homosexual for you?

Well, I had already come out as a homosexual. It was kind of a dirty mess for me.

Years before?

Yeah, although I'm not real happy with the homosexual community. Having AIDS kind of makes me feel like I'm a minority within a minority, so I'm feeling some of the discriminations of being a minority.

If you could pick one word that best describes your feelings, what would it be?

Handicapped.

Since you have become aware of yourself having AIDS, have you done any evaluations of yourself?

I have been to a psychotherapist and we've been processing quite a bit of things, a lot of stuff that I've had buried for years. You know, the fact that I'm gay, my self-worth and self-image, a lot of things.

How has AIDS changed your values about life and death?

I've basically discovered that I put the better things in life, you know, the really desirous things that I wanted, away for another day. I've had to take a look at that, and decide that maybe I'm never going to have another day. I'm not sure that I want to abuse myself with work, saying, "I can do this now and this now, and then I can enjoy things later." I'm really questioning that, although I haven't really succeeded at turning my life around. I think that I've stopped trying to invest in tomorrow, because today was really miserable.

Do you seem to be more in touch with your body than you've ever been? With what it needs?

I don't know that I'm more in touch. I think that more than anything else, I've been forced to be more responsible for my body.

How has your biological family responded?

They've tried to be supportive, but they're not dealing too well with my homosexuality. It's all kind of superfluous. Sometimes they seem more like a burden than they seem to be reliable, "lean-on" people. My brother and everybody have tried to be real generous and tried to be as helpful as they can. But then I don't feel that they're dealing with it very well. They think that if only I wasn't trying to be a homosexual, I'd be okay. They're not the kind of people I can turn to or depend on. I don't feel that it's their fault. I think the whole issue of homosexuality is the prime issue that they have, and that makes it impossible for them to communicate and to relate to me.

I can understand how the two together are just a little much.

It's very overwhelming.

Yeah.

I don't deal well with my family, but then I guess that's universal.

Well, it sounds like things really haven't changed all that much.

Yeah, somewhat. I mean, they've all sort of made a concerted effort to reach out and touch, which they weren't doing in the past. It's kind of like when I was a kid and was always there, but all of a sudden when somebody has a serious health condition like this, then they all of a sudden sit down and start getting in touch and stuff. The energy involved in that is appreciated tremendously. Even though they were very much in touch before, now it's kind of like slowed down. They're not maintaining.

What is your perception of organized medicine in the way they've dealt with this?

I think there are some very dedicated physicians who have done all that they are capable of handling and doing. I think that the A.M.A. politics has been hideous. Also, I feel that there are a lot of nonprofessional medical people who have not only overreacted to AIDS, but who have seen this as a mechanism to punish those people who are gay.

Yes, I agree.

I think particularly the A.M.A. has been shown up for the horrible, horrible policies of political groups that sometimes are less concerned about improving people's health overall, and more concerned with drug companies and their own self-perpetuation. Their ignorance and disregard for ultimate health care is clear in the medical treatments that we are receiving.

Exactly.

I'm really pretty clear that the medical practice has been caught with its pants down. But there are a lot of those doctors who are conscientiously trying to treat their patients, who are having to grapple with alternate health methods which are completely foreign to them.

What do you think about alternative treatments?

I feel that until the A.M.A. starts to acknowledge alternate health methods, we're not going to get the full health treatment that we need and deserve. And I think it's not just for the AIDS people, but I think it's for people in general.

How effective have psychologists been?

Well, I think that they have been thwarted in their world in this whole thing because obviously there's a lot of psychosomatic health problems involved in these things. And I think that an AIDS person is also a person whose health is definitely wrapped around the psychosomatic issue.

Do you mean stress?

Stress, and also the fact of our own homosexuality. I think we've built in self-destruct homing devices inside of ourselves.

I think AIDS is taking a kind of opportunity because the gay community doesn't have a very good self-evaluation.

How have psychologists helped or harmed us in that regard?

Well, they've not taken an active role in taking a fair share of the treatment of AIDS, and again, they have been thwarted because of the A.M.A.'s attitude about using chemicals. I think also maybe the therapist himself is still struggling with so many things that psychomedical work is something that they haven't delved into. But I really feel that because the doctor is so happy with his placebos, and with his authority, he really is the number-one thwarter of the issue involved here.

What about volunteer counselors? What's your experience been like with them?

I think that they have put together some of the most phenomenal people to ever be assembled to do these kinds of things. I have nothing but respect for these people.

And the gay community in general?

I think it's mixed. It's a slice of homosexuality that happens all around. Some are black, some are conservative, some are liberals. I mean, the whole spectrum is there, and all of the attitudes that are in the community at large are in the gay community.

What about the ministers and religious organizations?

Those people, I have nothing but loathing for. I feel that organized religion as we see it today has basically stripped away any opportunity for gay people to be religious what-

soever, except to try to build some kind of empire for themselves. I'm very disenchanted with M.C.C. [Metropolitan
Community Church] for the politics that they have, where
they've taken the church and made it into a personality clash,
as opposed to dealing with religion. I feel that the churches are
a justifying type of organization to destroy and hate gays.

What about the media? How has it handled this thing?

I think the media has played a very key role in discriminat-
ing about AIDS, allowing the homophobia, the thwarting of
the funding that should have been happening and labeling the
disease a gay disease.

Are you speaking about mainstream or gay media?

I'm talking about both, because I think that the gay media
has been no less guilty than the general public media. First of
all, I want to state that I feel that the media as a whole is more
interested in selling than in solving. I feel that the *Enquirer* is
more blatant than the average newspaper, but I don't find that
the other newspapers are much different from the *Enquirer*. I
feel that instead of informing the public, they've sold them on
horror stories and they have blown this thing to a much more
compromised situation than what it needs to be.

I would agree with that.

I think that not only has the media done a horrible disservice to us, but it's been a horrible disservice to other people
who are threatened by the disease.

**What about the federal government and the way that the
government has responded?**

The federal government is a reflection of the person who is in the White House. My feeling about the person who is in the White House is that he is not above using the CIA to "seed" the community with the disease in the first place.

You wouldn't doubt that?

I wouldn't doubt that and I'm real clear that he has no desire to cure or deal with this disease at all. It would be a real nice way to kind of, how can I say it, weed the community of fags.

So you think there's a political use for the epidemic?

Oh, I think that they're overjoyed about it! To the Republican and/or Christian Right, it's the greatest thing since Jerry Falwell got together and created the Moral Majority.

How will AIDS change the coming-out process?

I'm really chagrined that anti-gay people have made it into a punishment situation. Now that the disease has come about, they've been able to go into the closet and shake all the awful ideas and things that they think about gays. You know, it's kind of like saying, "If you engage in masturbation, you'll grow hair on your hand." Now the Christian Right is saying, "If you practice homosexual acts, you'll die."

6

One Day at a Time

Dan Turner

Dan Turner was the second man diagnosed with Kaposi's sarcoma at San Francisco General Hospital, early in 1982. A native of Bloomington, Illinois, he is a playwright and free-lance writer in his early thirties. Dan's first play was a musical for black high school students in Selma, Alabama, where he was a Vista volunteer. When Dan was interviewed, Cinderella Two, *his fifth musical, was playing in San Francisco. Dan is the public relations officer on the executive board of the People with AIDS–San Francisco political action group.*

I

When did you first become aware of the emerging AIDS crisis?

I guess it was the fall of 1981. I heard of it through Larry Kramer in the *New York Native*. In December I noticed my first KS lesion. Then it was gay cancer, or GRID—Gay Related Immune Deficiency. I was diagnosed in February 1982.

What was your prognosis, and what treatment options did you have then?

I was told I had cancer, that it was in my blood—systemic—and couldn't be cut out. I was told I probably wouldn't live very long. My doctor said to think good thoughts, deal with my problems. I did chemotherapy from March 1982 to July 1982. Then I was one of the first ten to do alpha interferon. I was a "star case" initially. Dr. Conant took me to Stanford in '82 for a demonstration; I pointed out my lesions and talked about myself in front of a group of dermatologists.

How were you feeling just prior to your illness?

I was in a state of depression. I was not happy with life. I was doing clerical work and I didn't know how I could continue in the arts. It was very difficult to sit in an office and type memos when I wanted to be creative. It was like sacrificing my soul for eight hours. My emotional life was unhappy. I wanted a lover, but the San Francisco life-style didn't seem to lend itself to monogamy. I did want to experiment, and eventually accepted that there was this kind of turnover. I accepted that this was the way of socializing and one could go along and enjoy it, or fight it. I remember when working at Bechtel I thought I would like to get sick, before I got sick. I daydreamed of being in a wheelchair, but being able to be creative . . . and that would be better! When I quit my job, the KS stopped.

Was your physical experience of the illness what you expected?

Not really. I've never felt ill, only inconvenienced by the treatments and being a guinea pig.

What did you do right after you were diagnosed?

Right after my diagnosis with cancer, I returned to the Castro and saw a musical—to cheer myself up. Then I went

home. The first housemate I saw was my oldest housemate
. . . he'd lived with me the longest. He cried. Then I phoned
my two brothers and told them. As I ran into friends, I'd tell
them if it came up. One guy fainted on the street; another
threw up. The effect was often that people personalized it—
they thought they could get it, too. Then they would freak.

**At the time, did you understand they were upset because
of their feelings of heightened risk?**

No. Someone told me afterward.

What emotional experiences did you have after diagnosis?

I had two big emotional releases during acupuncture.
They were related to discussing my spiritual crisis with a
straight therapist. I confessed all my sexual fantasies to him,
like he was my priest. I didn't feel good about fantasizing
about some of the weird things I thought about. I went
through a purging of my closet, so to speak, and I threw things
out. It was my way of getting rid of some of that fantasy stuff.

**Have your family members who know of your illness
made reference to your religious faith?**

My brother in Texas has become a born-again Christian in
recent years. When I told him of my situation, he wanted me
to start reading the Bible. We read the Bible over the phone
together. He sent me a Bible. I am a very spiritual person and
become involved when people start talking about those things.

**It sounds like you had your share of Christian guilt to
deal with.**

Yes! Having been raised Catholic, that's still something I
have to deal with. I am very tied up in that.

Did you reevaluate your life right after diagnosis?

Yes, I started doing it right away. When I saw I wasn't going to die in a week or two—that I have been given a reprieve, in fact—then I relaxed some. I feel somewhat secure. I feel a sense that there may not be a lot of time. My strongest desire is the creative desire to do the best I can in the time that I have left. Given the opportunities and resources I can put toward my music and writing, I'll leave my best. I live for my self-expression. But I love people, too.

An immediate conflict came up when I was diagnosed with AIDS. I was torn between writing something personal because I didn't have much longer to live, and something commercial to pay the bills.

I wrote a monologue, "Pearls of Wisdom," about the eighty-eight-year-old great-aunt of Adlai Stevenson. Stevenson grew up in my hometown and his great-aunt lived in my father's hotel. I used to interview the older people in the hotel who retired there, and the employees. So I wrote about her in the monologue. She is sitting in the hotel lobby, waiting for the doors to open to the dining room; my sister and I are playing with the dog in the hotel lobby where Grandma Stevenson is reflecting on her years of life. She is enjoying the passing of life even as she sits. I am thirteen—just coming of age. She is giving advice about surviving in life, throwing pearls of wisdom. I had a lot of respect for her, and somehow held onto her memory right after my diagnosis of KS.

When you were diagnosed, did you ask, "Why me?"

Oh, yeah. Well, the only information I'd heard up to then was that it was the sleazy ones who got it. I thought, "Gee, I could have been a lot more sleazy than I was!" I thought I had been too good to get this! I had been promiscuous, in the sense that I had gone to a few bathhouses. But I don't like to denigrate the baths because I don't think they are the problem. I didn't have "multiple anonymous encounters" or use drugs, anyway. I seldom even drink. I've never bought marijuana. I'd never done anything extreme like fisting.

What pulled you out of your spiritual crisis?

I released it all out. I feared that Christ might come in the room any minute. (They laugh.) I wanted a clean slate.

How do you feel about those issues now?

You know, I still have a problem with that. I still feel that it is very important to be resolved about these things . . . sexual things. I accept my sexuality, but I don't know how my sexuality fits with my ideal self. I feel it's okay to be gay—aspects of it. But what is proper sex? One crisis is between recreational sex and a relationship. If the church does ever okay homosexuality, it would probably hold relationships in a higher state of grace than just recreational sex, which they don't approve of. I believe there are worse sins in the world than recreational sex. I don't feel sex is high on Christ's list of things to worry about.

II

How have you evaluated yourself or your way of living since you became aware of AIDS?

With the knowledge of AIDS has come a fuller awareness of what it means to live in the present as opposed to the past or future. To take life a day at a time seems to be a worthwhile endeavor in itself.

In the beginning, immediately after diagnosis, I was more directly concerned with the status of my health, checking myself daily for new KS lesions. Now, after two and a half years, I feel more secure with my health and allow myself the luxury of forgetting the peril my body may face. I don't get overly concerned unless I feel run down or have a cough or temperature.

Recently, a new KS lesion appeared on my right thigh. It's small, but with it came the concern that a new bout with KS might be on the horizon. I realize that the threat is still present, but even though there hasn't been anything that obvious in two years, I plan to take the day-at-a-time approach and not get overly worried. Lesions have faded in the past, and I trust will do so again.

On the practical side, a diagnosis of AIDS is a reality and I have made several attempts to improve my attitude and daily habits. I make conscientious efforts to eat better, rest more, exercise, and relax.

I am more sensitive to the concerns of others, not as selfish as in the past, more likely to put myself out for others. I might tell people that I will say a prayer for them if they feel troubled. Since other people with AIDS have put themselves out for me, I feel good about sharing my experience with recently diagnosed individuals. I feel that I am a better person now because of my experience with AIDS—which at bottom is an experience with mortality.

In pursuit of goals, ambition and greed can begin to supervise our lives. With a genuine threat to the ego, values have an opportunity to reestablish themselves. I allow my spiritual side to venture forth far more frequently into the world.

Physically, I look better now, after diagnosis, than before, primarily because I feel better about myself. I am able to do what I like to do on disability. I am free to be creative. I felt trapped in clerical drudge work in the past and unable to express myself fully. I am not so driven as before. I can relax and work on projects at my leisure. I can take life at leisure, and not fault myself for impediments that get in the way.

If something bothers me, I feel free enough to let it go, not hang on to the frustration. Little things like being stuck on the transit system, or washing dishes, or taking time to talk or comfort others no longer get in the way. I simply take them in stride. I have learned not to fight with myself, but to let go of the frustration.

What sexual habits or preferences have changed?

Immediately after diagnosis I changed my sexual behavior. I had just ended an affair and decided to take a rest from sex until I knew the status of my health. I was concerned about giving CMV virus to a partner, as well as contracting another virus or VD from someone else. When I was told that I did not have an active CMV virus, I celebrated by going out one night and meeting someone. This was before we were told that KS was AIDS and there was such great concern about spreading the as-then-unknown virus. Exchange of body fluid was still questionable, so I was careful not to swallow. After that encounter there was more talk about limiting sexual partners and not exchanging body fluid, so I essentially stopped going out to meet people.

In the summer of 1982 I met a guy who lived in San Diego, and went to visit him twice. When I told him about my condition, he was not interested in sleeping with me. He was cautious to the point of not wanting to be in bed with me, but let me visit him because I was infatuated at the time.

During that summer KS and PCP came under the heading of AIDS for the first time and the media began to cover it more fully. I continued not having any sex during the period I was on chemotherapy from March '82 through July '82, and then through the initial phase of interferon in August of '82.

I met my boyfriend, Dan, in October of '82 through my

housemate, Bruce. He wanted to start a relationship with Bruce, but Bruce was not ready to be tied down. I waved my hand and said that I was ready for a relationship. He knew that I had AIDS, and decided to meet my doctors and give it a try, since he was attracted to me. He was very attentive to me and drove me to the hospital for treatment and took care of me when I had a bad cold, cooking for me at home. He lives in Oakland and has two jobs, so this was really putting himself out.

As the media attention increased and my boyfriend became familiar with some of the other people with AIDS, he began reacting on more emotional levels, along with everyone else, and became more and more concerned about his own health. He began taking vitamins on a regular basis and with far more conviction than I. He also became more concerned about our sexual contact. We continued having intercourse, using a condom, but less frequently. We stopped jacking each other off, because he was concerned about the cuts on his hand from his work as an industrial mechanic.

We continued having sex for the first year we were together and then stopped when I was diagnosed with a fistula and had to stop for a couple of months. We never started up again, and so have not had sex now for nine months. This has put a strain on our relationship. We still have strong emotional ties, but our temperaments are quite different, as are our working hours and interests, and now without sex we have little in common but our love and concern for each other—quite a bit in itself, but nonetheless difficult to sustain without sex and similar interests. I have started trying to go out socially more and meet some new people and this has met with mixed results.

Since diagnosis—two and a half years—my sexual activity, with few exceptions, has been limited to my boyfriend/lover, Dan, and an occasional j.o. session with myself or a friend. I still like men very much, and give them the eye when I am so moved. I have noticed that people's attitudes toward someone with AIDS have grown steadily more concerned; they are less likely to want to get involved, even so much as a date without sex. I have had a few dates to the movies. There is always a lot of hesitation when it comes to body contact, kissing, etc. Some people seem comfortable with j.o., but using a condom is somehow more risky—at least psychologically— than it is with a person not diagnosed. I tell people that it would be better to have safe sex with me than unsafe sex with someone not diagnosed, but that is still difficult for some to accept.

How has your view of yourself as a gay man changed?

The view of myself as a gay man has not really changed, apart from the fact that I must be more responsible in my intimacy with other men. I am still proud to be gay and feel good about myself and others who are gay. I feel that we will be a stronger group of men because of this challenge, and I hope that we can move forward and not let it shove us into despair. I hope that we can be good examples to gay men who come after us, and that they will still experience the inner freedom that we experienced, even though sexual activities have been curtailed.

Have your needs for emotional intimacy changed in your relationships with other gay men, gay women, and your family?

Yes, I do need to be intimate with gay men, gay women, other people, and my family and friends. There is the fact that time may be short for me, and that I'd better take advantage of all the relationships that I have and make each encounter worthwhile. The fact that time may be short has impressed upon me the necessity to make the most out of each moment I share with people in the here and now.

I took a trip back to the Midwest to visit my gay sister, my mother, and my brother in Texas a year ago, and brought my boyfriend along. It was a return-to-roots trip, a bit nostalgic. Originally, I had planned to tell my sister and mother about my diagnosis at the time, but after talking with my oldest brother in L.A. decided to continue keeping the facts a secret. My mother is seventy-six and we felt that it was still bad news and not something that she needed to deal with at this time in her life. My sister has an ulcer and did not need to hear bad news either. Since my health is basically good and I have no obvious lesions, it is not necessary that they know.

Have your beliefs about gay freedom changed any?

My beliefs about gay freedom have not changed. I think we will have to hold on to it more tightly now than before, because AIDS appears to be a threat to homosexuality, if not to the general public. The Moral Majority can use this disease against us and say it is God's plan or retribution, but theirs is a god of vengeance and mine is a god of love. Gay freedom must also mean gay responsibility. I believe we have rallied around the cause of health. We have largely had to fend for ourselves and support research and fund our own clinics. People have been slow to help us in many places. They have carried their fears of homosexuality into the health fields and media. We must defend our freedom as people at every opportunity. We must remind the general public that we are also part of the American democracy and government and our rights and health are just as valid as the next person's.

Have your values about life and death changed?

Life at best is brief, and a life-threatening illness can only make it seem more precious. To integrate the body, mind, and spirit in a productive whole has always been my goal. The main difference I have noted in my behavior is that I tend to act more for others and with more consideration for others now than I did before. With death from AIDS surrounding us, my friends, my community, my feelings of care and concern are broader and more inclusive than just concern for myself. I really care what happens to everyone else, and I admire their individual courage.

There have been many fine examples of bravery from the beginning. It is ennobling to see how fellow gay brothers have fought off the horror of progressive KS and debilitating PCP, have won and gone back to work and then had to fight it off again. In the midst of physical struggle, some have also waged political struggle for the gay community at large. They have shared themselves for the benefit of those following after, and this proves that they held their gay freedom very dear. It is really an honor to continue the fight for them, each other, and ourselves.

Death takes on more meaning depending on how you lived your life. I like noting that gay men are strong men—especially emotionally—they are very caring men, and are not afraid to hug and hold on to one another in crisis. I would doubt that the love would flow as easily between other groups of people. Perhaps we have already been an example to those who do not understand our sexual persuasion. At least they can see the love we have for each other as people.

Has your ordering of time or your experience of time changed any?

My ordering of time leaves room for the weather and the little things of the day, the dishes, the cats, the garden, a walk down the street, the casual small things. I take more time with time. In some ways everything has equal value. I do not attach more importance to one moment than to another. Each is important, has meaning and value. Quality of life happens, I think for me now, moment by moment, not periodically.

How has your biological family coped with AIDS?

I told my oldest brother, who is the head of the family, that I have AIDS. I also told my next older brother, but did not tell my mother or my gay sister. My oldest brother and his wife sent me about $1000 to help with bills my first year of diagnosis. I talked to them on the phone. My oldest brother donated some blood for research at one point.

At the beginning they reacted to my diagnosis with cancer as I did. I have sent them information in the mail on AIDS as it became available, and also some reports and interviews with me that were printed in the paper. There was interest and concern, and all was kept between us. They have seven children.

The family at large, such as my aunts, my mother's sisters, was not informed. We have really kept the news from most of the family. My brother and his wife have been supportive on the periphery. They do not call regularly to see how I am doing. They assume I am doing well, or I would call them.

My brother is practical and not emotional. He has not involved himself except when asked. My other brother in Texas has had emotional problems in the last few years, and has primarily given spiritual support. He has not written. In the beginning we talked on the phone, and he recommended passages for me to read in the Bible, which he had sent my sister and me shortly before my diagnosis. I am sure he includes me in his prayers, and he has been spiritually helpful, giving me some tips on my visualization work.

My sister is aware of AIDS, although she does not know that I have it. Recently, a gay rights ordinance was turned down by the voters in Duluth, Minnesota, where she lives, and she sent me letters to the editor to show me how homophobic people were. Among them was someone who was concerned that homosexuals would move to Duluth and spread AIDS to the general public via drinking fountains.

My mother was aware of the AIDS problem very early,

before it was called AIDS and was only known as KS. She warned me not to get the disease the very Christmas before I was diagnosed (in 1981). I actually had the first two lesions at the time she warned me. Mothers can be intuitive, and since mine is also well read, it did alert me to the fact, and was instrumental in my taking as fast action as I did to get the initial biopsy.

How does allopathic medicine define and treat individuals and the symptoms of AIDS?

Allopathic medicine treats AIDS symptoms, not the disease itself, so there is a lot of fear and doubt attached to the many treatments that have been tried on people with AIDS. I have had five months of vinblastine chemotherapy and two years of alpha interferon. I have not experienced any bad side effects with either treatment. Vinblastine was low in toxicity; my hair did not fall out; I was not nauseated.

I did go sterile while on the drug, but am now fertile again. Because of that I put my sperm in a sperm bank, since I was concerned about becoming permanently sterile. I explained to the doctor that it was an assumption that gay men would not want to have children. I have a close writer friend who has fathered a child, for instance. I might want to do something similar later in my life.

When interferon was made available to ten of us at San Francisco General, I decided to try the experiment. I wanted to go off chemotherapy, since interferon was more natural to the body. I was selected to do low-dose interferon, and have done well on it, and am now the only patient of the original study still doing the dose. There is a question as to whether it is actually working, but it's presumably helping in some capacity. At least I have not had any major colds or flus—virtually none—since I began two years ago. A new lesion has appeared on my leg, but we will have to wait and see whether it will be a real threat or not. One must maintain one's attitude and general health at all times with AIDS.

How does mainstream medicine relate to government control of AIDS?

The government determines what is officially AIDS and what is not. The CDC has defined KS and PCP and some other opportunistic infections as officially AIDS. The government also had to give approval for Pentamidine for PCP up until recently, when it was accepted in trials. Drugs, experimental and otherwise, and protocols and companies are monitored by the government. I believe there do need to be requirements for new drugs. At a time like this, though, it is important that research not be inhibited, and that the testing not be detained by red tape.

I believe that health care is in the general interest of the public and that the government should see that no one is denied health care or coverage and that adequate space be provided for those in need. I would support a national health care program or socialized medicine, as long as research was not inhibited or red tape slowed everything down more. The health of society must be protected and minorities in that society should not be isolated and made to bear the burden of an illness. Those that stand in the way of AIDS research are only hurting themselves.

How does homeopathic medicine define and treat individuals and the symptoms of AIDS?

Homeopathic medicine treats the whole body, the mind, the spirit. I got in touch with this at the same time as I went the traditional route. I have faith in all those who try to help. I do not exclude traditional doctors, nor do I exclude those practicing alternative therapy. I have made good use of both medicines.

I began acupuncture at the same time I began chemotherapy in March of '82. I feel that I had some good results with acupuncture. It has helped me to relax and get a sense of body balance, alignment, energy. I feel that it helped stimulate my immune system. It was also important that I feel that I was doing something for myself, as well as others doing something for me. I had acupuncture once a week the first year of my diagnosis, during the time I had major medical coverage with insurance. A year after termination from work, I lost my major medical coverage and had to begin paying for acupuncture myself. This has made my visits more infrequent. I went about once a month for a while, and in the past year even less. I have worked out a payment which is not too bad, but does not allow me to visit once a week, as before. In some ways this has been a test to see just what kind of good it was doing. Now that I have a new lesion I am more concerned about reducing stress again, and so would like to start being more regular with my visits to the acupuncturist.

I also began taking large doses of vitamin C at the same time I was diagnosed. This eventually became about twelve grams of C a day, usually in a pill, sometimes in powder form. I also take a multiple vitamin, a B-complex, sometimes extra zinc, evening primrose, lecithin, and L-Orinthine, depending on whether I am visiting my boyfriend in Oakland. Usually a multiple, twelve grams of C, and a B-complex are enough for me.

I also consider regular exercise homeopathic, and have kept up my occasional running and weight training. It makes me feel good and look better, and that is important where health is concerned. One's attitude is better if one feels and looks better. At first I didn't push myself a lot, and took things at a comfortable pace on the different treatments, but now I don't baby myself quite so much. I push myself more and feel that it is good for circulation. When I'm tired I stop.

How does alternative medicine relate to traditional medicine in practice?

I have not had any problems with doctors advising me against alternative therapy. My doctor says try what I think will be helpful. Fortunately, the protocols for interferon have not been so strict as to limit other choices such as vitamins, exercise, or acupuncture. Time is involved in the practice of both medicines, and suspicions have developed in both fields of the other, but I think the best attitude to have is that each is trying their best to help and that the patient should not begin with a bias toward either.

I have never been discouraged, but rather encouraged to try other ways of helping myself. Because of that live-and-let-live attitude and not exclusionary approach, I have a much better attitude to those doctors who practice traditional medicine. I think that each side should have a healthy respect for the other.

How does alternative medicine relate to government control of AIDS?

I am not aware of what kind of money the government spends on research in alternative therapy. I would hope that it provides in some way, since so many people have found it beneficial and worth investigating.

The doctor who originally diagnosed me with KS believes in holistic health, and his entire approach with me was one of total body response. How am I feeling? How should I try to improve my whole outlook on life, physical, spiritual, and mental? Through him I had the right attitude to approach some alternative therapy on my own and not be afraid of helping myself, not just depending on "the experts" or the traditional doctors.

How would you characterize the effectiveness of psychologists and volunteer counselors in dealing with the AIDS crisis and PWAs [Persons with AIDS]?

At the beginning I steered away from psychologists and volunteer counselors. I wanted to get a handle on the crisis myself. I wanted to see what I could do for myself first. What kind of control could I bring forth? What kind of responsibility could I muster up for my own disease? I think it helped me face it first. I listened to advice when it was offered. I decided not to see a psychologist, but to talk to friends, relatives, or doctors when I had questions. Eventually I attended a support group to check in with others to find out how they were doing, to compare notes. I found out that I could be there for them and give comfort to others who were more concerned about their health and less in control. I found the turning outward helpful not only for them but for myself.

Eventually I took volunteer counselor training, did some role playing, tried to develop some listening techniques so I could be a better counselor in my own right, working on a local AIDS switchboard, which I initiated and volunteer with weekly.

How would you characterize the effectiveness of ministers and religious groups in dealing with the AIDS crisis and persons with AIDS?

I have a friend who is a priest who administered the sacrament of healing the year I was diagnosed. I got in touch with my spirituality by attending church shortly after I was diagnosed, talking to the minister and members of his church. I found the energy very high there, the singing, and met some people with physical challenges who were doing well and had good attitudes about life. I also began expressing my spirituality in my visualization work, helping to relax my body through spiritual imagery.

It was recommended by a man who studied Chinese medicine that I express myself freely and not hold anything inside that could stagnate in my system. I began to express myself publicly in forums inside meeting halls and out on the street at rallies. I spoke on the radio and television and was interviewed in a feature TV show and for local gay newspapers. I became active as a person-with-AIDS on the board of a local AIDS organization from its inception through the present. I continue to serve as a member of another AIDS organization as well as the representative from San Francisco and People with AIDS on the board.

This has taken me to other cities to health conventions as a participant, actively involved in the fight against AIDS. I have spoken in New York, Denver, Minneapolis, Dallas, and Seattle, as well as in San Francisco, and participated in articles or talk shows out of town.

All this work has been therapeutic. It has taken the fear away from me and given me a sense of accomplishment and control as opposed to loss and failure.

How would you characterize the effectiveness of gay and mainstream media in dealing with the AIDS crisis and persons with AIDS?

The media has sometimes played up the sensational aspects of AIDS and sometimes been afraid to show the truth. I completed a public service announcement to be run on television with three other people with AIDS. Evidently it was difficult to get the announcements on the air because people complained about a guy putting his arm around another guy in one case, and in two of the announcements the visible lesions would have offended people.

After the media challenged one AIDS organization for moving too slowly with some of the education campaign, we find that the media is reluctant to help us spread the word more plainly. Part of the checks and balances are because people are still afraid of the effect of homosexuality on the general public. Homosexuality is still more feared than a disease like AIDS itself.

Evey gay media took its time the first year, because I think they were concerned about the effect AIDS would have on gay businesses. Now they are better at keeping up with the latest information, not afraid to do feature stories on men with AIDS and put obituary notices in the paper.

How would you characterize the effectiveness of the federal government in dealing with the AIDS crisis and persons with AIDS?

The government has been slow to fund all possible grant requests for AIDS—as discussed at meetings of an AIDS organization. Proposals should be considered carefully, but some have gone begging because of government red tape or cutbacks.

How would you characterize the effectiveness of the gay community in dealing with the AIDS crisis and persons with AIDS?

I am aware of changes in attitudes toward AIDS in the gay community primarily through my gay housemates. I have seen them become more aware and concerned since they found out that I had KS. At first they were slow to take it all in; they dealt with it as a diagnosis of cancer. They did not feel personally threatened. It was not clear that it was being spread sexually at first. Then there was the attitude that it would not or could not affect them. This has grown less and less clear and, with each additional case, of more concern.

As people hear of more and more friends coming down with the syndrome in one of its forms, they too become more concerned for themselves. They are more likely to practice safe sex and be cautious about keeping themselves in better health. My housemates decided to buy a dishwasher. Some use disinfectant more regularly in the bathroom and are concerned about specific pans I may use to wash out my eyes. I use hot salt water for my eyelid infection, blepharitis, which is probably immune-related.

I have started going out socially again, and notice that people cruise less directly. If the subject of AIDS comes up, they are more likely than before to lose interest in me as a prospective friend or companion. People can only take so much bad news.

Individuals as well as gay businesses seem to have a threshold for how much AIDS talk they can take. Most seem to cooperate with posters, flyers, and brochures. Some hold benefits, have cans to raise money, or put up posters. Many try to keep business as usual. When the National AIDS March was held in October of '83, Castro bars were reluctant to put up the posters in their windows for fear it would turn business away.

I helped develop the safe-sex poster with two naked guys which said "You Can Have Fun—and Have Safe Sex Too," thinking this would be more appealing and catch the eye. It did seem to work; at least people were more likely to put the poster up and take notice.

The gay community has already responded quite well in San Francisco to the AIDS crisis. We feel that the education and information have reached a lot of people because the rectal gonorrhea rates are way down, which is a good sign that people have been paying attention to what we have been saying. The community must find new ways of relating sexually, and in some cases the old way must give way to the new way. J.o. clubs have become more popular as it has become necessary to close the baths for want of a way to monitor existing unsafe sex behavior.

Last night I spoke at a forum for people with AIDS. We

discussed the sociological and psychological problems of being a person with AIDS. Although it was raining, the turnout was pretty good and everyone stayed to listen to what three of us had to say. We introduced ourselves and told a bit of our personal history. Then we explained our medical situations and talked about treatments we are doing or have done, both traditional and alternative. We spoke about dealing with AIDS psychologically, how we told our relatives and friends. In one case the fellow said he explained he had AIDS to his parents first, before explaining to them that he was homosexual—which appeared to be a more difficult subject for him to broach with his father.

I think the gay community respects people with AIDS quite a bit. Bobbi Campbell did a lot for our image right from the beginning of his diagnosis in September 1981. He wrote a column in the *Sentinel* gay newspaper explaining a lot of the things he was going through at the time. This coverage was early and very good. No coverage was going on like it in the *Bay Area Reporter* at the same time. He helped explain the syndrome and his tests and treatment to the public, and dealt with it bravely and realistically and not sensationally for them. He was an articulate, rational voice for the community and set a good standard for future PWAs. Several other PWAs have spoken openly and honestly about their fight, including myself over the past few years.

Personalizing the disease has gone a long way to dispel some of the myths that have cropped up, such as the idea that persons with AIDS were people who trashed around a lot, did drugs, fist-fucked, etc. Certainly some of those things have applied in some cases, but I believe a clearer image of average-Joe gay being susceptible to the illness is now present.

At the beginning I felt compelled to get the message out with the doctors that AIDS threatened the entire gay community, not just a certain portion of it. I think that has now been accomplished. Now, the question addressed at last night's forum is how to live with AIDS. How does life go on? How do people with AIDS have dates, have relationships, have a quality life? How does the rest of the gay community live side by side with people with AIDS? Can they give them the kind of support that they need?

It is hard to get close to something you fear. Other gay men are now being asked to rub shoulders with people with AIDS, to get close to them, to like them. This is a difficult task. As people fear AIDS, can they still like and love the person with AIDS? That is the question.

I approached a popular gym to see if discounts could be had for PWAs, but my idea was turned down. The gyms want to "stay clean." They are afraid of the bad effect on business. People with lesions are thought to be a detriment to the gyms. Questions have been asked about sharing hot tubs with guys with visible lesions, etc. There is an attitude that if one has a beautiful, muscular body, one will not get AIDS or one does not have AIDS. This is unfortunately not the case. Bodybuilders have come down with AIDS, and going to a gym will not prevent guys from getting AIDS—only safe sex will prevent AIDS. Once a guy has AIDS, he may still go to a gym and work out—the exercise may still be possible and good for him, and he should not be discouraged from doing so just because he has a few noticeable lesions. If his doctor approves of the exercise, then the gay community should let the guy feel welcome.

PWAs have encouraged safe sex behavior by helping to write pamphlets, brochures, and posters. Laws that single out specific places as dangerous are not particularly effective. For those practicing safe sex, the closing of the baths is an infringement of their rights. Better perhaps is a big sign that says, "No lifeguard on duty. Swim at your own risk."

The gay community must not hide in the closet on any issue, including AIDS. We must continue to insist on money for research and quality health care, and support relief programs. Many would like to shove AIDS under the rug, in the closet, like families used to hide retarded children or whisper about their homosexual son or daughter.

The nation now knows that gays exist, and also that gays get sick like everyone else. We must not be embarrassed about life and death matters. We must show our support for all those afflicted with AIDS and rally around their individual causes. If we deny our own people, then the future sanity of boys who want to come out will be jeopardized.

The AIDS epidemic is only an advantage for the Christian Right if we cower and let it be. Our attitude should topple theirs by virtue of Christ's example of caring for the sick. He didn't go around Galilee trying to change people's sexual persuasions.

7

Speaking for Ourselves

Bobby Reynolds

Bobby Reynolds is a man in his thirties who lives in San Francisco and works as a PWA health-care advocate. He worked for a public utility company before his illness. Bobby is on the Executive Committee of the Persons with AIDS–San Francisco action group. (An interview with Bobby's lover, Mark Wood, is presented in Part Two.)

I

When were you first aware of AIDS?

It's kind of hard to remember exactly, but I think it was in the winter, maybe, of '81. That was from articles I had read in gay papers.

When were you diagnosed?

The doctors diagnosed me officially in June of '82, but I had diagnosed myself in March of '82.

How did you do that?

It's just—I saw the spot on each of my ankles and just knew what it was.

And between that time that you diagnosed yourself and the doctors diagnosed you, what did you do for yourself?

What I did was try to cope with the information I didn't want to acknowledge, so I sort of pushed it to the back of my mind and gradually got up the courage to show Mark, and I said, "Look at this flea bite I scratched." And then a week later I said, "You know, it's funny—this hasn't gone away." That was about as far as I could go with Mark, and then I went to the doctor and I said, "I want you to look at this spot—I think I know what it is, but I don't want you to tell me it is, because I haven't had all the fun that those guys have had." By that time the stereotype of promiscuous, fast-lane—and so, on one level, I was knowing all along what it was, and I just was having a hard time.

Had you had any other kinds of illnesses before, like six months to a year before you noticed the lesions?

That was real interesting—that year was probably one of the healthiest I'd had in a number of years. I ended up carrying sick leave over from '81 into '82—so I don't remember carrying very many illnesses at all during that year, the prior year.

So this whole notion of risk—risk for contracting the disease—you don't seem to feel that people who are in the fast lane are maybe the most apt to get it?

That's an interesting question. I think I will respond by saying that from what I have heard and learned over the past few months and years, it seems like the more sexual contacts you have, the more likely you are to come in touch with whatever agent it is that seems to give your system this AIDS. So I guess, using that definition, the more "promiscuous" you are, the more likely you are to be exposed to it.

So that's the way you would define risk? In this case, as multiple partners?

It's hard, it's real hard. There's more than one thing involved, and it isn't just specifically sexual contacts. I think that your body has to be in just the right depleted state from stress, from anxiety, from not enough nutrition, from maybe too many drugs, like prescription drugs or recreational drugs. So I go for the multifactor sort of theory that there's more than one thing involved. And then this agent enters the picture, and that's it.

From your own experience and your self-knowledge, what is your experience of your illness?

Little purple spots that the doctors say are there because my immune system is not functioning properly. A little white spot on my tongue that they say is common when the immune system isn't functioning. Some parasites and things that are in my intestines that they say are there because my immune system is not functioning properly.

Has your own definition of risk had any effect on the way that you dealt with yourself after the diagnosis?

I have a philosophy about life that I've had for a long time, even before this happened, and there are certain things that happen to a person in his or her life that allow that person to grow and stretch and become better, let's say, and I think that this, AIDS, has happened to me for some cosmic reason. I'm not really sure why. I don't really spend a lot of time thinking about why it's here or if it was because I did this or that or the other thing, but it's in fact here. So now I'm dealing with it, and I'm trying to do the best I can. Does that answer your question?

Yeah, but in terms of the treatments that you are involved in, what treatments do you do?

I have been taking chemotherapy since August of '82.

What kind of chemotherapy?

Vinblastin twice a month.

So this was just outpatient?

Outpatient.

This is just an injection you get?

Right.

And what kinds of vitamin treatments or things like that do you do?

I take some multivitamins, and I have for years, but I don't personally have a strong belief in high vitamin treatment. I have tried biofeedback and found that it works for me, and I tried visualization and I find that it works for me in terms of stress reduction.

When you visualize, what is it that you visualize?

We're talking about Pac-Man. The first time I was exposed to visualization was at a support group. In 1982 there was another man with AIDS there who asked me if he could lead the session. It's quite common to close the support group meeting with that, but I didn't know. He said that if you could close your eyes and hold the hand of the person next to you, imagine that there is a white light entering your body, and the

white light is Jesus and your body is the temple, and the bad
germs or the cancer cells are the moneychangers that Jesus is
chasing from the temple. So I figured, okay, I could try that,
and I closed my eyes and I saw Pac-Man chewing at what I
imagined were my cancer cells.

What did the cancer cells look like?

Little round fuzzy discs, sort of, discolored. I can't even
remember what color initially I saw them as.

How many Pac-Man eaters?

Initially, there was one. Of late, I send armies, and I sur-
round myself in a glowing green light, and inside that green
light are millions of Pac-Men just sort of doing their stuff. If
we're talking about somebody specially who's not there or
somebody who's in the group, I imagine their bodies covered
with this light, with all my Pac-Men in it, or I shoot little beams
of Pac-Men to where they are.

How are you doing with the illness?

Very well, physically, mentally, and emotionally.

**How would you describe your emotional experience with
AIDS?**

The beginning, I remember a slight sense of disbelief, like
this wasn't really happening to me and I was watching a program on TV and the fine tuning was out of adjustment. Everything was a little fuzzy. There were times that it was just like
—I'd be talking and I'd forget, I'd blank out, I couldn't remember what was happening. There were times that I'd sit

and shake. Numbness; the first couple of weeks were that. I guess up to actually about eight weeks, that went on, feeling a little scared. There was a lot of unknown at that time.

Gradually as I got some questions answered and went through the staging to find out my physical condition, some of that fear started to dissipate, and some of the numbness went away, and the anxiety level sort of lessened. I quit work after about a month—I took a leave. And as the months wore on there was this sort of change. I decided to make some adjustments and I decided to do things, and I became more confident about what was happening, and I was becoming more in charge of what was happening to me, so that I was becoming stronger physically as well as emotionally.

Looking back on it from this point, it seems kind of strange that I had that reaction, because I've become pretty well in control of things now. It's not that things don't upset me. When they do, I find that I sort of take a couple of days that are real quiet and go off by myself and process it internally, and then I allow myself to start talking about it in bits and pieces to people, and then I can vocalize.

Does it seem like you're, in fact, more in control of your survival than ever?

Yeah, yeah, the reality of it was they said I was going to die. My experience of it has been that I'm not, *but* there are still those statistics out there that seem to indicate that most of us do die at one point. The reality is that because we're born, we're going to die.

Life is terminal.

Exactly. So I feel in a way that they've given me this gift, and they've allowed me—whoever "they" are—allowed me to do things in my life that I might not have done had I just left, you know. Well, someday I'm going to die, so they've given me sort of a period of time to deal with that.

Do you have as much choice in terms of being public about being homosexual after you're diagnosed with AIDS?

Whew! I kind of feel like that decision was taken away from me at one level. There just wasn't anything being done to offset those stereotypes and those labels that people were putting out there, that all people with AIDS were gay and they all had this and they all had that. I felt that they were putting me on a file card and just sticking me away somewhere. So I made the decision to start speaking out, and I became known as Bobby Reynolds, the person with AIDS, and consequently they're going to know that I'm Bobby Reynolds, a gay man who has AIDS.

So I feel in a way like that was decided a long time ago, and I didn't necessarily think about that consciously when I was starting to do what I did. Looking back, in one respect it's funny, because we've talked in group about how coming out with AIDS is similar to coming out of the closet as a gay person: a lot of questioning, a lot of trying to find your identity, who am I as a gay man, who am I as a gay man with AIDS? It's like crawling—starting out in diapers and then crawling, then standing up, then taking your first step, and it's very similar, I think, to what people go through coming out.

Have you noticed any changes in any particular behavior since you were diagnosed? Life-styles, behaviors?

I think I've become more selfish, allowed myself to be more selfish.

Self-preservation kinds of things, you mean?

Yeah, I give myself strokes. I ask for strokes when I need them. I don't do things because somebody thinks it's something I should do, but I do things that I want to do because I want to do them.

Is it easier to say no?

Yeah—yeah! It's okay to say no, too.

What about your needs for emotional intimacy and hugs and things like that? Have you noticed any changes?

I have always been an emotional, touchy sort of person, and that was sort of different than the way most people are. I find that that's been heightened in myself, except that now I'm surrounding myself with people who react the same way— they're emotional and emotionally accessible. Not that they're emotional all the time. You know, sometimes they're right underneath the skin. There's a lot of huggy people around Shanti, and around the clinic, also.

Have you noticed opportunities? I mean, we talk a lot about the dangers of AIDS, and it really is a life-threatening illness, but what about opportunities for intimacy between men with sexuality changed, diffused? Have you noticed a lot of opportunity for intimacy?

It seems like it cuts down a lot of barriers, being diagnosed.

Barriers for intimacy?

Barriers for all different levels of interpersonal contact. I never would have thought that I could sit in a room with a man that I didn't know and talk about my deepest feelings, and not feel afraid to do that, or that I would be able to sit there and hear someone else talk about that, or that I could reach out a hand and touch somebody when they're hurting and know I helped, or vice versa, they could do the same to me. Society sort of conditions you to put up barriers.

In terms of your attitudes toward society and these attitudes toward barriers to male-male intimacy, what have you become more aware of? I mean, you've already said this has sort of heightened your awareness of that, but what are the implications for our gay community and for society and us learning this intimacy?

I think this is awful to say in one way, but I think that AIDS can be a great educator if people really listen with their hearts, and a lot of people have. I've been amazed at the number of people that have been caring and supporting.

I think that I try, whenever I can, to help people find the humanness in themselves, that they maybe had lost touch with, and to relate to me as one human to another rather than as a gay man to a straight woman or whatever label you put on it. I have a lot of hope that by doing that, myself and all the others that are involved, one-on-one, we'll be able to help make changes. I think it's going to be a slow process, but I think that unless you take that first step, you won't get anywhere.

II

During the time shortly after you were diagnosed, did you do any self-evaluation to figure out where certain personality traits you have, certain images of yourself came from?

Before I was diagnosed, I went to a psychologist for a number of years because I was in trouble dealing with a medical condition called hypoglycemia. I had been able to treat it by regulating my diet, but at the time it caused depression and anxiety and anger. I also had some things from my family that I wanted to deal with and didn't know how. He helped me find the tools within myself to work on those things, so I addressed a lot of that well before the diagnosis and got to the point where I like who I am.

So you sort of picked and chose from among all of these sources of your identity and emerged as an individual that accepted yourself?

Yeah, uh-huh.

How has your experience with AIDS affected your values about life and death?

That's a rough one. I don't know that I allowed myself to think much about that before diagnosis. I just was—you know, you went on and you planned stuff and you didn't have much death in your family, hopefully, or in your daily life. But I've been put in touch with my own mortality, and that's kind of scary. I don't consciously spend a lot of time thinking about it. I've gotten to a point where I just—I tend to live, day to day, and do what I want to do and how I want to do it. And dealing with dying, well, I don't know if I've dealt with the possibility of my own death, really. I have intellectualized about it, and I've talked about it, but the reality isn't there, so I don't know how that's going to be.

What's been really difficult is seeing so many men my age and younger die. Getting to know them intimately, and I don't mean in a sexual way, but just getting to know them and watching helplessly as they fade and die. That's a bitch.

Have you made a will?

A will was made before diagnosis. Mark and I bought property in Colorado, and we decided at that time to draw up a will and agreement. I forget what else we did—there was like a living will and power of attorney. Things like that. So that was dealt with several months before I knew I had AIDS.

How would you describe your encounters with or your analysis of people in the social systems or institutions that you've experienced, like, for example, your family? How effective and supportive have they been?

My family is basically all dead, except for a sister, some cousins, and a great aunt. My sister has been a shit; that's my natural reaction. The reality is that she's afraid, and I can understand that, and it hurts that she's not being able to be there for me.

Where does she live?

Daly City—about twenty minutes away. It frustrates me that I've tried really hard and—I tried really hard to help her. I've been able to help a lot of people, and she like shuts the door in my face and she's the one I want.

What about health-care providers and organized medicine? What is your perception of what's going on there?

My experience has been mostly wonderful. There have been a few cases where I have learned to become an advocate for myself and told someone to fuck off or not allowed them to touch me to take blood because they always bruised me or something. But I really have had good experiences. You don't hear that shared by everyone, but I've had good luck.

What about psychologists and counselors?

Some I like, some I don't.

Tell me something about the ones you like. You don't have to mention names, but in terms of what they're saying or writing about.

What I really like about them is the fact that it seems like they really hear what people with AIDS are saying and they are responding as if they have heard.

Are these mostly gay psychologists who live here in the Castro area, do you think?

I don't know where they live, but I think they are all gay ones that I am thinking of.

And what about the ones that are writing things that you don't think are favorable?

I have some problems trying to stay open to them. It seems like they are unable to go from their head down into their heart to relate to people. They deal with people with AIDS in a very clinical, sterile sort of fashion, and a lot of them have agendas: "You are this way because you sucked off twenty-nine people on the twelfth of such-and-such a month." They come in with a mindset that doesn't allow them to stay open or to explore other realities.

What do you think about pre-AIDS personality work?

In my nonprofessional little life here, I think that it's a lot of baloney. It really upsets me that—that—it's like trying to be fit into a square peg, and I'm a round hole—you know what I mean! It's like they're trying to fit me again on this file card, that part of me fits. But I'm me, first and foremost, and I think that you have to look at each one of us as individuals, and some of us share things, and some of us don't.

How would you describe your encounters with ministers or religious organizations?

Very minimal, really. I've spoken at a couple of forums where there have been ministers or religious lay people. I really haven't connected with a lot of them.

How does Jerry Falwell's position make you feel?

That jerk! It's someone using religion or using politics or using whatever for their own—it's like he's got a mindset, and so he's going to do whatever he can to fit gay people and AIDS into his mindset and justify his mindset however he can. God didn't put us on this earth with these feelings and—you know, it's crazy, it's crazy. I also feel frustrated. Just me—in speaking out for myself, I have effects on those that hear me, but he's got national coverage. So I feel that I'm in this big lake, and he's got this big tidal wave coming at me. It's a little overwhelming at times. That's how I feel about the psychologists, too. A little overwhelming.

Do you think Jerry Falwell's going to heaven?

I'd like to make a suggestion about where he'd go, but I think that the decision is taken out of my hands.

How about the media, both mainstream and gay? And let's start with the mainstream press.

Near and dear to my heart, this topic is. I've had a lot of contact with media. It was kind of fun, to begin with. Then it became more of a chore, and then it was back to being fun, and it's all just mixed up together now. The problem with the media is that they are not set up to deal with emotions, unless it's rigged somehow. If it makes their point or their story, that's fine, it can be included. But otherwise it seems like it's not appropriate to have on TV or in the papers or whatever. I think they really lose track of the humanness of people.

What about the gay press?

There are some members of the gay press that I hold near and dear to my heart because I think they've really dealt with my life and the lives of my brothers in a very sensitive, caring way, and then there are others in the community that seem to have blinders on. Again, this mindset, it's like they have to justify the position that they've taken, and they see it as a power position sort of, in many cases.

This is probably the most interesting aspect of it to me: the power that's involved. Clearly, we're all men. I mean, the movement has been dominated primarily by men, and the media has been dominated by men. It seems like there's a new game in town, and the power struggles that go on seem to be geared to diminish the power that might be achieved by these emerging leaders.

Which emerging leaders? People with AIDS?

Yes, the people with AIDS and spokespersons for AIDS—does that ring any truth to you?

It does, yeah. It's like, again, going back a couple of years:

We started speaking out for ourselves, and I think for a while we were heard, but now it's all these people speaking for us as if they were us, in many cases. I don't know. A number of us have tried to reach them on a one-to-one level, and it doesn't seem like it's working.

How do you think the gay media could be more effective?

I think my answer applies to both gay and straight media. They have an incredible opportunity with AIDS, what's happening with AIDS, to educate and sensitize all segments of communities. And instead, it's go for the sensational headline, go for the quick story or front page, or go for the Pulitzer, and most always it's to the detriment of somebody.

What about government statements and government funding and regulation? What's your impression about the government and how they're reacting to this epidemic?

I'm real skeptical. My experience with the government was rejection two, three times for Social Security benefits and reading in the papers, "Well, we *are* responding—we have appropriated millions." But then I'd hear from the doctors and the people "in the know" that all these appropriations were sitting there and they had not been released. So it's like the government was lying. I haven't been able to get away from it. I still feel like they've lied and cheated.

And the gay community—what do you think about that— their response? First, maybe, I would like you to define what you mean by *gay community*—what your thinking is.

My initial reaction is to think of that sort of five-block-square radius where I live—the Castro—even though it's more than that. I guess the response is on a one-to-one level. I've seen people react to me individually and on a larger scale—the gay politicians, the gay health-care givers, the gay support givers, the gay businessmen, the gay you know, I'm not sure exactly what I really mean by *community*. It's kind of a perception that you have inside your mind, and it's kind of hard to put into words. It's all—the people you see in the paper, it's the people you see on the street. It's the guy next door, and it's the Democratic Club—and it's hard for me to give you a specific on what my gay community is. It's a lot of things.

Well, then, let me just ask you how you feel the gay leaders have responded to the AIDS epidemic.

A lot of them have been less than adequate.

Do you think that they feel like it's just really a fly in the soup, a turd in the punch bowl, and that's just a real bad thing for their job?

My sense of it is that—and this isn't all of them—there are some that really care, straight and gay politicians, but the gay politicians see AIDS as being an opportunity to grab on to an issue, either for or against, you know, there's both sides. For me, it feels like they've taken my life and made it a football, and they're tossing it back and forth for their own betterment, or their own glory, or to make their point, or to get extra signatures on a petition for their cause or something. It seems real impersonal for a lot of them.

How do you think the AIDS epidemic will change American culture?

(Pause.) I don't know how to answer that. I have hopes

that it does change. I can't fathom this happening to people—this awful thing happening to people—without some good coming out of it. I think on research levels that the research into AIDS could open doors to other types of cancer or other types of problems with immune systems or any number of things. I think that the government could learn a lot from this. I don't know if they will. I think everybody could learn a lot, and I don't know, again, I don't know if it's going to happen.

What's the most important lesson that could be learned?

The first response that came to mind was that people are people. You know, we're not file cards and we're not labels and we're not stereotypes or statistics. We're people, and we breathe, and we hurt, and we bleed when we're cut, and we have fathers and mothers. We are people.

How do you think that it will change the gay movement in particular, especially if we broaden our scope of humanity and achieve this revolution or renaissance, I would say, a humanitarian renaissance?

I see a lot of positive growth, and this is a guy that's not been very politically aware or involved or anything. But certain things have changed, so I have to be more aware of some things, and I see a lot of growth in the gay political arena. I see a lot of unities coming together on all different levels to fight for a common purpose. And I think that can only be good, in the long run. It will show that people can work together, that you don't have to have this group and this group and this group separate, but you have one large group with a number of different participants.

Do you think that what might be able to come out of this would be a legalization of relationships?

Whew.

Will this assist us in arguing that gay relationships should be legalized?

I think that we have the opportunity to display the validity of our relationships to a broader audience now than perhaps before, in a different way, and I think that it could help, but I don't know if it will.

If that were to happen, what would be the implication for gay culture?

I think that relationships with significant others would be validated no matter who they were, that my lover would have the same rights as my mother or father or sister or wife, or whatever, in legal matters, and would be as accepted in social matters as if I were married to a woman.

Will we still have gay ghettos?

My gut reaction is yes. But not necessarily for the same reasons as now. I think we band off in ghettos for protection. I think if certain things are taken away that we may be able just to band together because it's fun. Sit amongst your own, like that.

What kinds of roles within the family structure could we play if we were to broaden our scope of humanity? Could we have a "Gay Uncle Day" or a "Gay Lesbian Aunt Day"? A national holiday, an institution in the family for those of us who choose to be with lovers of our own gender?

God, that's a really nice thought! The way the world is

now, the way this country is, I don't see that happening for many years, but, God, it would be really nice to be validated that way.

Are there any tips that you would like to offer to people, either with AIDS or the people who are now being called "worried well"?

To be gentle with yourself. You know, don't beat yourself up if you can't do what you think you can do, because things change. Um—I guess that was the important thing, be gentle with yourself.

Thank you.

You're welcome.

PART TWO

Gay Family Network

8

A Stronger Pair

Mark Wood

Mark Wood is the lover of Bobby Reynolds, a gay man with AIDS whose interview appears in Part One of this book. Mark works at a gay restaurant in San Francisco.

I want to talk with you a little bit about how your awareness of AIDS evolved. When did you first become aware of AIDS?

It must have been at least two years ago, because I'm pretty sure that I was reading the articles that Bobbi Campbell was writing in the *Sentinel* newspaper. He started in the fall of '82; I was reading those for six months, and then there'd be other AIDS-related stories in the other local gay newspapers. But it wasn't until May of '83 when Bobby was diagnosed that I *really* became aware of it and I learned a lot.

Before your lover was diagnosed with AIDS, had you met anyone with AIDS, that you knew of?

Not to my knowledge. I only knew of the couple of more well-known people in the city. I'd known who they were. I had never met them. They weren't acquaintances of mine. I just knew who they were, and I knew of their struggle with it. But no one personally.

How did you think of your own risk of contracting AIDS at that time?

Almost nonexistent. I never, at that point, thought that it would be the remotest possibility. Because at the time they were telling us that it was the people who lived a fast life and did lots of drugs and had multiple sex partners and took part in a lot of kinky sex that might endanger them. I didn't fit any of those criteria; I didn't feel that I was too susceptible. I'd always been real healthy. I'd never had any lengthy illnesses other than the standard gay diseases of VD and some strep throat, but never anything that had debilitated my body for any period of time.

How long had you and your lover been together?

We've been together almost five years now, so at that point we were together for three years. We met in April of '79, and I guess this all happened in May of '82.

How did your notion of risk change after your lover was diagnosed?

Well, it was never clear, and it still isn't today, obviously, on how one contracts AIDS and how it's passed along and who's at the most risk. I figured that I still was at a very low risk because neither of us were taking part in any of those other things. That is, until the doctors made concrete statements like, "We're limiting you in your choices of what you should do sexually and limiting the number of anonymous sex partners that you have," and having what they later referred to as "safe sex" and stressing a real healthy diet and sleep.

When I realized that all of those things were necessary, I realized that I was pretty much abiding by all of those things anyway, so I felt my risk never increased a whole lot, other than the simple fact that I have been living with a man now for almost two years who has the impaired immune system. Why he got it, how he got it, why it doesn't go away and get better or clear up by itself is very puzzling and, at the same time, I suppose I have to ask myself, "Is my exposure to him on a day-to-day basis over a two-year period—is it likely that it would impair my immune system as well?"

And have you noticed any changes in your health?

Not in my overall health, but after going through some of the tests that are being offered to lovers and friends and significant others of people with AIDS, I've been made aware that my immune system is somewhat suppressed, which is not untypical of a gay male in a population of people here in the city or anywhere. We do tend to have suppressed immune systems, and mine happens to be one of them. I'm aware of that now, whereas two years ago I wasn't aware, because nobody was aware. They weren't doing studies and they weren't giving that information out to people that it's kind of a normal thing that gay men will have a suppressed immune system. So now I'm aware of that and I try to keep that in mind.

Why do you think gay men have a low immune system?

I have no idea. I mean, if the doctors won't even come up with a suggestion, I'd be the last one to start trying to.

Sure. How has the whole AIDS crisis made you feel, on a real personal level?

I guess we've gone through a lot of different things. The disbelief about it happening to someone that I love so much and who is so important to my life, the hurt that it was him and not anybody else—why him? The anger at seeing it change his life so much and then seeing how it ruins and takes the lives of people that we've become close to. That's really frustrating and it's maddening and then, throughout it all, there are wonderful, supportive people and there's always hope.

You have to be optimistic about everything that will come tomorrow and the next day and with more research and more dedication and more care. There are wonderful support people out there that are making life easier for all of us. If we ask for that help and support, it's out there.

I've gone through a lot of different emotions and feelings about it, and I try to stay on sort of an even keel so that I can be a steadying, supportive base for Robert, so that when he has his real down, unhappy, unpleasant times—they're more frequent for him because he's the one that's dealing with it and he's the one that's closest to the other people that he sees in clinic visits and in the hospital and hears about their latest bout of sickness.

How has it changed your relationship?

Well, I think that we're probably even closer now than we were before. I think we're a stronger pair. I know he's a stronger person individually, and that makes me feel real good to see him grow and become a much more outspoken and courageous and caring person. When you stop to think of all of those things, it's really admirable. I think our time, when we spend it together, is more beneficial to us both. There's less clutter in our lives.

It sounds like you have cut out the bull and gotten down to the core of what it means to have a relationship?

Yeah, and friends that we had before and that were acquaintances that you used to spend time with or think about or want to fit into your busy schedule, you know, some of those are no longer important because they've made the choice, too, for whatever reasons, that they're not needing to be in your life. That's fine, and there have been a number of other people that have replaced them, and they're the ones that are directly involved in the crisis that goes on each day.

If you could offer some kind of tip or advice to lovers of people with AIDS, what would it be?

Well, it would be different, of course, for every situation, for every two different people, but I think probably you just need to be real supportive and be someone who will be there to listen. Sometimes that's all you can do and sometimes that's the best thing that you can do, is just to be there to listen and put your arm around and give him a big hug, and hold him and not try to tell him it's going to be any better or say, "It's not that bad." All you need to do is just be a caring, loving person there to listen as they sort of unfold the traumas that are going on.

How has AIDS changed your notion of what coming out is all about?

Gee, I don't know, I haven't thought about that, but, my lord, I think that it would be—young kids today coming out would probably have a lot of fears and a lot of second thoughts about "How soon do I need to take this step?" and "Should I stay in the closet a little bit and not fool around and not explore my own sexuality?"

It's quite possible that that's happening to a segment of the sixteen-to-twenty-year-olds, or twenty-five-year-old, group of people in our country, because the things that they read and the things that they hear are certainly enough to—anybody with a conscience, not necessarily a brain, but certainly a conscience. But then you really can't expect or demand that of them when their older, more seasoned and mature peers who are in their thirties and their forties are not listening and taking the advice that they should be gleaning from what they read and what they hear from their doctors.

If they would take the opportunity to go to some of the forums where they could get educated and ask any questions—when older people in the community aren't doing that or they're doing it and then not listening and continuing some of their ways that might be detrimental to a healthful life or a longer life or a safer sexual experience for them, then you can't blame the younger people for not following those examples.

Sure.

So it's got to be difficult. I guess it's not something that I have thought of myself, since I've been out for a while, and it just isn't something that I've had to deal with myself, but I would imagine it's kind of scary.

Have you changed personally from the whole experience of AIDS?

I don't think so. Our relationship when we met was somewhat more open, and that was mostly because of my work situation, which took me out of the city for periods of time. It was sort of agreed that whenever I was away, I was able to function as I would want to and when he was living at home here, he was able to carry on. To a small degree, he did that, and to probably a little bit of a larger degree I might have, when I was away.

And then when I stopped working on that job and being away—that was the first two years—then the third year of our being together, I was home all the time and it was understood that we just weren't fooling around with other people, unless we did it together, unless it was what you call a "three-way." And that happened rarely. He would have liked to have had more of those experiences, he says. He always maintains that he'd like to do that more often, but very rarely would he pursue it, so I couldn't take it too seriously. I never felt that I needed to be the one to procure anybody. If he wanted something like that, he could introduce it into the situation.

So we were pretty monogamous all of the time and it's like you must and you need to, and of course I know that there are a lot of wonderful men out there and lots of wonderful bodies and lots of wonderful, easy, and anonymous sex could be had, and is had by most gay men who walk around on the streets. I often think that I'm missing something, but on the other hand, I know that it's not worth the risk, not only to myself, but to Bob.

That's one of the first things that was really missed out of the whole thing about not wanting to see AIDS people out and about and being in bars and being at baths, because they were afraid that they were going to give it to somebody. Well, in fact, the bigger risk was for the AIDS people themselves, that they were going to get some kind of a virus or a disease or a flu from something that would weaken their system.

So, yeah, I know that there's a lot of happening things out there and I'm content not to be a part of it, because it doesn't make any sense. I mean, it will always be there and in years to come it will be there for us or for me or for anybody.

So your relationships with other men are more intimate but less sexual, is that fair to say?

More intimate, yeah.

In your relationships with other men, do you find that you are more supportive and touching without sexuality?

Oh, yeah, definitely. I guess maybe I'm able to be more

understanding and supportive of some of my friends. I might not have been able to be a year or so ago, mostly because I'm learning to be more tolerant and less judgmental. I was talking to one of my friends the other day—Bobby and I have both known him for four or five years—and we mentioned that someone was doing an interview with us about couples who have a connection with AIDS, and he said, "Well, maybe it's about time that somebody did a story on the vast number of single men out there who are in the situation of being concerned and trying to live healthy gay lives and yet safe and still having sexual relationships, and what it is for them to be going through as well."

One of the greatest things for us is that we've had each other throughout all of this time, and we have had one another to hold and rely on and count on and have sex with and stuff like that, but for a lot of single men, they don't, and it's real difficult for them. And so I'm real understanding when I hear my friends talking about their dating habits and their patterns and their unhappiness with striking out and not finding the one true boyfriend out there for them. It's difficult, I know.

How has this affected your values concerning life and death?

When you're young and healthy, you don't think of dying. I mean, you're not supposed to program that until you're sixty, seventy, eighty, or something like that, and now that I see it happening around me, I'm much more aware that it's a possibility. It's come too close too many times in the last year or so. It's taken some wonderful lives and cut them off much too early.

So what do I say about that? That it's not right, that it's unfair—there's no explaining it, and why won't it end? Why can't we find some reason and explanation for all of this and put an end to it? Because it shouldn't be happening. And I guess I have a healthier respect for it and a closer understanding about death, and because I do, I think I have a better appreciation for every day that we're all alive.

How has your family reacted during this period in your life?

My family, since they've been aware of Bobby's illness, have been real good. I didn't tell them right away about this. He was diagnosed in May. I probably told them about nine months later in a letter I wrote to my parents. I had told other members of my family who live closer to me here in California much sooner than that, and from the very beginning they were very understanding and supportive.

The bulk of my family who don't live anywhere around here and wouldn't necessarily have ever found out about it—I mean, it could have gone on indefinitely, but finally I felt that it was important for them to know what was going on with the most important person in my life. I wanted them to be aware of what he was having to deal with every day and I wanted them to be enlightened.

I wasn't ever asking for sympathy or anything like that, but I just wanted them to know that I had something of great concern to my life and that perhaps I was going to be less accessible to them and I might be more preoccupied and I might not be able to do things with them in mind. I was more concerned about taking care of my own home here. But they understood that and it was fine, and they're always questioning and wondering, asking how Bobby is, and they sent cards and support in the ways that they know how, and it's been a real good learning experience for them. They seem to show quite a lot of concern about it and want to educate themselves as well, so I've been real happy with them. I think Bob has, too. He's gotten a lot of good feeling and support from them, as he's probably told you he didn't get from his own flesh and blood.

Uh-huh. What about health-care providers? How effective do you think organized medicine has been in dealing with this?

I guess the overall picture is not wonderful. It's been a good two years, three years now, probably. Some people even say the first cases were as far back as '79, and that makes it almost five years in some of these cases that people have been dying from it, so when you stop to think of that, five years is an awfully long time for all these questions to be hanging over our heads. When you consider what modern medicine and technology has to work with—and there are those who would say that some of that responsibility falls on the government for not releasing funds soon enough and getting concerned enough about it quickly enough, and that they are at fault for not speeding along research and trying to wipe it out. And I would have to agree with that. There's an element of that.

So you feel angry that the government has not responded?

Sure. You have to feel angry when you see the people who waste away over a period of months and years and die because there's no good treatment and lots of different possibilities. It's not a pleasant situation to be going in, and God, how frustrating it is, hearing about the things that people have to go through with doctors and with the insurance companies and getting their medical bills taken care of and squared away and companies that they've worked for being totally shitheads about it and not being understanding. Yeah, it's frustrating and we'll never know how many lives could have been saved if treatment had been administered immediately and more research was done faster.

What do you think about the way the gay community will change as a result of this?

Or will they change?

Are they changing?

I think last year, around the time of all the news stories when the media hit it real heavy for a while, people did lighten up and stay out of their traditional playgrounds and probably got a little bit better rest and laid off drugs and drink for a while. As much as I could tell, most of the people that I knew did that, and I think too many of them, the vast majority, did it only for a short period of time and now are feeling that they can return to those activities. I mean, it's the only thing that some of them ever knew, the only way to relate to someone was through bathhouse sex, anonymous sex. Some people had such low opinions of their own self-worth that they let themselves be abused sexually and mentally, and unfortunately, I think they'll always be that way. I don't think that a crisis like this is going to change them overnight. I don't know what or if anything ever would, really.

But there must be a segment of the population out there who have heard all of the awful things and have been able to sort through it and picked out the facts and then related it all as much as they possibly can to themselves, because it has to be different for each and every person. I mean, you can't make a blanket policy or statement that would be effective for everyone. I think that the thinking and caring ones are making those decisions and are going to come out of this a whole lot better and a whole lot stronger. There's going to be an awful lot of pain for everybody involved before that happens, but how that will be demonstrated, I don't know.

The people who were saying last year that it was time to settle down and become monogamous and find a husband and all that silly stuff—I'd be real interested to see how many did. You'd like to think that a lot of them did and would and are still out there working and sacrificing and giving up their Saturday nights at the baths or their Sunday afternoons or their promiscuous sex and lots of drinking and drugs. I'd like to think that some of that was happening and that they would start feeling better about themselves and learning to live for themselves and with themselves and by themselves. You have to do all of those things even if you have a lover and are in a relationship. You have to be able to do all those things anyway, and what better time to be learning how to do it? If you stop to think about it, it might be a wonderful time for people to be preparing themselves for real good relationships. I guess that's a possibility.

It sounds like the thing that perhaps we've all learned is that recreational sex isn't just for fun and that we can't just objectify ourselves and other people like we were animals, but in fact all sex affirms us. It affirms our core character regardless of whether or not we're aware of it on a conscious level. All sex is affirmational.

Oh, yeah.

How do you think this gay epidemic will affect society at large?

I'm not sure. I guess it will make a difference if it ends real soon and if it doesn't spread any farther into a larger gay community or into the general population as a whole, because I think if it did that there would be a lot more unpleasantness and ugliness directed toward the gay community. So for everybody's sake, it would be wonderful if all this would end yesterday.

If it continues to grow and gets real nasty, who knows how it will change people's life-styles? Probably people will put forth theories about rounding up gays and keeping them segregated and penned up and all those awful kinds of things that some of those right-wing moralists would just love to see happen. But I don't think the crisis is ever going to get that out of hand or that the country as a whole would ever condone something like that happening. I'd certainly hope not.

That wouldn't be a pretty sight if that were to happen.

9

A Mother's Love

Gertrude Cook

Gertrude Cook is a sixty-two-year-old woman who works at the Oregon State Ombudsman's Office. Her son, David, died of AIDS on October 3, 1983. Gertrude was caring for David when he died in her arms.

When did you first learn of this new disease, AIDS?

It was early in 1982. We knew that David wasn't feeling well, and then Fred, his good friend, talked with me about AIDS. When David became more ill, I became very aware of it.

So your knowledge about AIDS came primarily from Fred?

Well, primarily from Fred, and there was a group of friends. David lived in a remodeled Victorian, and it's kind of like a small community. Somehow the illness wasn't very insidious at first, because it didn't apply to me personally, or David. But then, as he began to get weaker and began to show signs of not feeling well, then I became very interested in it.

Uh-huh. Did you know that he was gay before this?

Yes.

Without using the term *AIDS*, how would you describe his illness?

Well, at first he lost weight quite rapidly. He was always concerned about his appearance, and he didn't want to get too heavy. Then he lost about thirty pounds without any explanation for it! I was real concerned, and then he told me that his lymph nodes were swollen, and then about that time I became aware of AIDS. I read everything that I could find about it.

What year and month was this?

Let's see. This must have been March of '82.

When was he diagnosed with AIDS?

He was never really diagnosed with AIDS. His doctor was very careful not to say that he had AIDS. He had Kaposi's sarcoma and Burkitt's lymphoma with underlying causes, probably AIDS, but it was never really vocalized. Well, it was, too. It was an insidious disease, and David wanted to keep it from me, and I wanted to keep it from him, I think.

Did you talk very much about it with him?

Well, yes, we did some. He refused to believe that he had it, and that might have been his downfall. But maybe it was the thing that saved him—saved his sanity. He always thought that he was going to get well.

Uh-huh. Did you think that he would get well?

In my deepest heart, I didn't think he would; but, of course, I hoped that he would. I was afraid he wouldn't.

Yeah, I understand. . . . Do you know that I have AIDS?

Yes, in your communication you said that you did.

Okay, good; I just wanted you to know that I'm real sensitive to what you both have gone through.

Well, it was an experience. Lon, I thank my stars that I was lucky. I'm very fortunate that this surgery I am now undergoing didn't come along when I was trying to take care of David. It would have been tragic. I'm glad I had the resources and was able to go down and take care of him. I think it was kind of good for both of us. I don't know what kind of relationship you had with your folks, but David and I have always been very close, and we've always had fun together. He liked to have fun. But we developed a respect, I think, mutual respect that we hadn't had before.

That's wonderful!

Well, it really was wonderful, and I think that no tragedies can happen without something of positive value coming out. I made some very special friends throughout David's illness that have become part of my family.

How long was he ill?

Well, let's see, he was only *really* ill, maybe the last year.

And he passed away when?

The third of October, last year, '83.

How did you perceive your own risk for becoming ill with this disease?

I didn't even consider the possibility, Lon. Well, from

what I've read, and I am not that familiar with the disease, I think that body fluids are probably the main way to transmit the disease. In the hospital, and when I took care of David, I took normal precautions. I wasn't so foolish as to not disinfect myself after I had taken care of him. I took normal precautions, but I was not in the least bit worried, and I'm still not concerned. My family was a little bit concerned when I got sick that maybe I had contracted AIDS, but it didn't even enter my conscious mind. I wasn't at all concerned about it. There was no question in my mind that I would take care of him if he wanted me to. The risk factor wasn't even considered.

The next series of questions has to do with your emotional experience. How has the AIDS health crisis made you feel?

I feel that the government should allocate unlimited amounts of funds to find the root of it. I think it's an insidious disease. They found Legionnaires' Disease without any problem. They've found other diseases, and I think this is no different from that. I feel very strongly that large amounts of money should be allocated for research.

Uh-huh. What one word best describes your feelings about AIDS?

One word? No, there are two. Sad and frustrated.

Is there anything about your son's death and the moments just before and after that you would like to share?

David died at peace. He loved life, and he didn't want to die. He died in my arms, and I think he was afraid of being alone at the end. David's cousin was there—my nephew—and his family, and David's doctors. Steve's uncle was there, and we had a home health care nurse that we became very fond of, which created a bond that will never be broken. It's something that's priceless to me. I did all I could for him. I think David had a fine life. He loved life. He had a good time. It was tragic that it ended so soon, but it was an enriching experience for me. It's a tragedy to lose your son and probably the worst thing that could ever happen to a mother or a father, to lose a child.

We've never talked about his father.

His father and I separated. His father makes Archie Bunker look like an angel!

Oh, no!

Yeah! He really is. It was very, very difficult for David's father to accept David's life-style first of all—and then to accept his illness! In fact, his father said to me, "I don't think you ought to go down there among all those people." And then David's thirty-sixth birthday was the nineteenth of September—he died the third of October—and so they had a birthday party for David. Sixty or seventy of his friends! We just brought him home from the hospital, and they came to visit him. We had a hamburger fry, a barbecue. David's father and his brother and family came down. I wasn't sure how David's father would accept him, but, you know, I was very proud of him. He accepted, and he circulated among "all those people." He had said "those people," but they became persons to him. He doesn't talk like that anymore. It was an experience. It was probably a broadening experience for him as well.

How effective do you think your own biological family was in dealing with this?

They were very supportive. My sisters were very supportive. One sister came down—I have two sisters—after David died, and we closed his apartment. They helped me pack his things, and his father came down. David's brother came down. His brother is seven years younger than he is, and his name is Steve. Steve's wife is a nurse, and they have two children, Abbie, who is four, and Justin, who is one year. They came down on David's birthday and spent a week. They were very supportive of him. David was always one of our favorite family members. All of my family feels very supportive. I haven't had any hassles.

About organized medicine—how effective do you think they've been in this crisis?

They were excellent. I couldn't have asked for kinder doctors at the hospital. Everyone from the X-ray department, the emergency room, the intensive care, the nurses on the floor that took care of David. There was never any reticence. There was never any hesitation. We never were made to feel that we were outcasts.

What about psychologists? Did you have any contact with psychologists?

Psychologists—the only person I was upset with a little bit was when David was home, somebody from a university—he was doing a research paper on AIDS victims and how they lived. He came in and asked to have an appointment with David and said that it would take an hour. Well, at the end of two hours, I went in, and they were very upset with me, because I was interrupting their talk. I felt that David needed to eat, and I was rather upset with the man. The man was rude. Perhaps he had a job to do and needed as much information as he could, but that's the only sour note of anything that happened.

What about volunteer counselors?

We had a fellow who, as I said, became part of our little family. He's just a dear, dear person and a dear friend, and was so helpful. He worked during the day at the hospital—or worked regular hours to make his living—but then he would come over. He was a nurse, and the fellow next door was a nurse, and so with their expertise they helped me turn David and do the things I couldn't do for him. Two women lived downstairs, and one of those women was a nurse who helped me, and the last five days of David's life, one of those people sat with him during the night so that he wouldn't be alone. So that was how I could get some sleep.

How about ministers and religious organizations—did you have any contact with them?

No. I'm not particularly an atheist, but I didn't find any solace in religion. They did not reach out. They're turning their backs on AIDS victims. I think it stems from the old original concept that the gay life-style is wrong in the eyes of religion.

Yeah, I think you're right. What about the media? How do you think they've handled this?

Oh, the media can't be blamed, really, because they have to search out news, and after something's been around for a long time, and even though there are many, many deaths from it, it seems to be newsworthy.

Earlier you mentioned federal government; is there anything else you'd like to say?

Well, I think the federal government should have the main responsibility in funding research for AIDS victims and to find a cure for AIDS. I think that's their responsibility! They have funds they can release for research and funds that are allocated for research and must be used for that. I think we need to make our political leaders aware of the fine, *fine* people who are contracting AIDS. There has to be something done to cure it! I feel very strongly about that.

How do you think the AIDS epidemic will influence society's treatment of homosexuality?

I think society sees homosexuality as some foreigner. I remember that my family used to say, "Oh, those damn Italians!"

(Laughs.)

And then we moved across the street from an Italian family and found that they were fine people. And the same way with blacks. My husband, he's still very much opposed to blacks. Collectively, maybe society looks askance at a disease or a life-style. If you can know the people individually, and they become individuals, then that's a whole different ball game. My concern is that so many fine people are contracting the disease, and there isn't anything that we can do about it. We need a program to find out what the cause of it is, and find out how to cure it.

How do you think that AIDS should change what the gay movement is doing?

Well, I was very heartened to learn San Francisco is making it easier for people who feel they've been discriminated against because of their life-style as gay or lesbian to file complaints. I think that's something the gay community can focus on. My feeling is that we live and let live and that I have no right to inflict my beliefs on someone else. What we do in our homes and in our bedrooms is nobody's business but our own.

Do you think that AIDS will change the whole notion of coming out for younger people who are not coming out?

I think so. I think AIDS has made people aware of a gay life-style that maybe they haven't been aware of before. I think that as we progress in our society, hopefully we can get this feeling that you can do whatever you want to do as long as you don't inflict your views on someone else, if they don't want to be influenced.

Do you think that there's a potential for the Jerry Falwells of the world to turn this into another McCarthy era, even more oppressive toward gay people?

Well, we're always going to have those people. Again, this is a free country, and I think we're always going to have some people who follow emotional issues, right or wrong. I don't think you can counter those kinds of people with any kind of valid argument.

Has this changed your own feelings or your own values about life and death?

Well, yes. I had never in my life seen anybody die. It certainly made me aware that it's something that we all have to go through, and it isn't something that needs to be violent. It was very beautiful, as a matter of fact. It was something that I will never, ever forget. I think the people that were there will never, ever forget that feeling of peace and tranquillity and special bonding.

Is there anything that you'd like to say—for history— about this?

Well, I will always be—I don't know if angry is the word—resentful, perhaps, of a society that would allow a disease like AIDS to get started and to continue and not find a cure for it. That's something that I will always carry with me. I feel that David's life was not in vain, and I promised him that we would always remember him. It probably has made a better person out of me. I think I'm more considerate. I know that I've been able to visit my friends in the hospital and to talk with them about death, when I never could have before.

I tell you, I'd sure be proud to call you "Ma."

Bless your heart.

10

He Was My Brother

Jerry

Jerry is a self-employed building contractor living in North Carolina. He described himself to me as a thirty-four-year-old, 210-pound, six foot-one-inch heterosexual man in perfect health, who hopes to become a millionaire. Jerry and his wife have two children. When Jerry's brother became ill with AIDS in San Francisco, Jerry came to his brother's side. This self-declared "white-middle-class WASP" from a conservative Southern community brought his gay brother home to live his last days surrounded by love.

What do you consider important to who you are?

I am married; I am a father of two girls. I'm a good guy. I am the median-average person. I am white middle class; like the old term, I am a WASP. A white Anglo-Saxon Protestant.

When did you first become aware of AIDS?

Probably in 1981 or 1982.

What was the source of this knowledge?

The television. Not locally. It's a whole white Anglo-Saxon Protestant community I live in. If you needed people for a movie that was to be set in 1933, you could come to the town I live in and find them!

Isn't it amazing that it's 1984 and we're still producing children who believe like pre-Depression?

Yeah, it is, but then, if you talk to the parents, you can understand it. I have met more ignorant people in North Carolina than anywhere else that I've been.

You've lived in other places?

Yeah; I'm originally from West Virginia, and I've lived in Ohio for a while. Well, now I'm in North Carolina. But I've found more ignorant, just stupid people in North Carolina.

What do you mean?

It all goes back to the education level. Every place that I've been before emphasized education and going to college. In the particular section of upper North Carolina I live in, there's an emphasis on dropping out of high school. It's understood that people drop out of high school in this area. They don't have a very high ratio of graduating seniors going on to college. It's sorry.

What was your first contact with a person with AIDS?

My brother. I can't actually figure out if he really knew he had AIDS or not. Yet he told me that he was in his fifth year. But then, this was almost at the end of his life that he told me that, because of things that he had seen over the past years, after they told him. I also believe my brother had a death wish.

Really?

Oh, yeah, a strong death wish.

For how long?

For all of his life.

What are your age differences?

I'm thirty-four; he was thirty-eight last December. So there were about four years. But just growing up and observing him, I saw the death wish was always there. The suicide wish was always there.

Did he ever make a suicide attempt?

I think he did, but he would never really tell me about it.

So he was hospitalized for one?

Yeah, that I know of, but I think it was for something else, but again, I'm not really sure. His idol in life was Marilyn Monroe, this tragic woman.

Well, our lives as gay men are pretty tragic because of our romantic pains; I can see the identification in this way.

As long as I can remember, she was his idol.

Do you know any other people with AIDS?

No, I do not. When I was searching for someplace to take my brother to, I found out that in the Greater Tidewater Virginia area there's only been maybe a half a dozen reported cases of AIDS, and it's extremely difficult to talk to anybody who knows anything. In the medical field it's extremely hard to find anybody who knows anything at all, or who has treated a case. What they were telling me was that usually the cases were being individually handled in this area by the family doctors. They just didn't know what to do, and there just weren't that many cases.

What do you think the doctors do in cases like this?

I think they just give drugs. Well, actually, I think they just try to make it easier, because they don't know what to do. They don't have any kind of background knowledge. They can't go to that many journals to find out what they *can* do, so they try to treat the symptoms as they show up. Doctors just use strong antibiotics and tell AIDS victims to avoid people who are sick themselves. They just try to "family doctor it" how they did it in 1900, because they just don't *know* what to do.

How close were you to your brother before he got sick?

Well, he was living in California and I live in North Carolina. So, when you talk on the telephone and you write letters, you write other things and talk about other things.

How often did you guys write?

Really only on major holidays. I have little children and he worked for a publishing house and he was very interested in books and wanted to get our kids on that track, too. He used to send them books and Creative Playthings toys and there'd always be a note and all. Then we'd either call or write a little note back. It was just off and on. I can't really put any kind of a frequency rate to it.

When was he diagnosed?

I would say six months ago. He died February 26. His last day of work was November 12 or 13. He told me that last May he was in the peak of health. Last June he went in for tests and I guess in June everything fell apart. Growing up, my brother was five-foot-eight, slight build, the original ninety-eight-pound weakling!

Did he have problems with health?

No. In fact, he was always much stronger as far as being healthy than me. I was always the sickly little kid.

When he got a sickness, he didn't get sicker than most people might?

He never got sick, I was always the one who got sick. But, at any rate, the story goes on. After he got to be about, I guess, about twenty-three to twenty-five, he became interested in bodybuilding. He put on a bunch of pounds and trimmed out his muscles. He looked extremely athletic then.

Was your experience of his physical illness what you expected it would be?

No. I could not believe it! He spent two weeks at Thanksgiving with us, and left, I guess, the first week in December. At that time I figured he'd lost some weight, but no big deal. Sometimes people do when they're sick. At that time he wasn't sure whether he had cancer, or whether he had AIDS, or whether he had something else. He called me about three days after Christmas, and told me that he was going into the hospital, after giving it a year. He went in the third of January and they released him on the twenty-fourth; he came here to us.

I couldn't believe it, because we had put a thirty-eight-year-old guy on the airplane in December. When he came back in the end of January, there was this little old sixty-five-year-old man they brought off the plane. I started crying, I really did. I went to the airport alone to pick him up. I didn't know what to expect, and when I saw him, it just blew my mind. His doctor in California had tried to tell me, but there's no way you can say something like that over the phone.

His doctor takes care of a *lot* of AIDS patients. From what he said and from what my brother said, the two of them really hit it off, and I guess my brother was this doctor's favorite patient. After my brother came here to stay with us, I spoke to his doctor about two or three times a week, just to say, "What do we do now?" The doctor had been trying to find for us somebody on the east coast to take my brother to.

He had quite a lot of friends, and a lot of people were writing to him and all. The ones that I could call, I did. His wish was to be cremated. We had these little "In Memory" cards made up. And the people that I couldn't get in touch with by phone, I sent them the "In Memory" cards.

That's very nice. When you took care of your brother, did you worry ever about what your own risk for getting AIDS would be?

The doctor from San Francisco said to use more common sense than anything else, and we just approached it from that aspect.

How do you think that persons with AIDS are at risk for getting other infections?

Oh, it's tremendous. If I had AIDS, I would hate to be around any little kid, because little kids are notorious for sicknesses.

Right. (Chuckles.) And everyone seems to think that the risk is the other way around—that the child is at risk.

Yeah, but that's because people are stupid.

How do you control against catching AIDS? When you were taking care of your brother, what kind of common-sense measures did you take?

We kept things antiseptically clean. We washed soiled linens as quickly as possible.

What would you recommend to people who are in your situation, in terms of how to take care of someone you love who has AIDS?

Try to find somebody who's been in the same position and talk to 'em. AIDS is not known whether it's transmitted by a virus or whatever. So we took the measures that we could against bacteria. If it's transmitted by a virus, well, you can't take precautions against a virus because that's airborne. The thing about AIDS being sexually transmitted that is kind of crazy is that, if it's a virus, it doesn't matter.

How do you find somebody to talk to? I'm always aware of things, and if you think that there's something—if you think there's an agency, a person, or something—if you think it ought to be there, it probably is. You just don't know how to get ahold of it. So you just have to try to get ahold of it.

What do you think the government should do to prevent AIDS from spreading?

I don't know that the government can or should get into it, because when you get into the bureaucracy, you never know what's gonna happen and you don't know if finding a cure won't be stalled for ten years.

Yeah. What do you feel about people's reactions to AIDS?

The vast majority of the people panicked when there's no reason to panic. If you say "AIDS," they automatically cringe and they say, "Oh, no!" And there's no real reason for them to do that, which again is because of the stupidity of the majority. And, I don't know, if you could do anything, it would be bet-

ter education, because that's the key to everything. I kept asking, "What's somebody else done that's been in my position?"
I felt I wanted to keep trying to take care of my brother.

Why did you take this on?

Because he's my brother. He was my brother and he
needed help.

How did you feel about him being gay?

It's his life, not mine.

Did you feel that way even before he became ill?

Sure. I live my life; I don't expect anyone to listen to me. I
live my life my way. I don't want somebody telling me how to
live my life. You live your life your way. You don't want somebody telling you what to do. If we don't try to force each
other's ideals on each other, we can live and let live.

**What emotions have you felt toward society's reactions to
the AIDS epidemic?**

I'm mad as hell, because the majority are so stupid!

**If you could educate all of them, what would you do?
What would you tell them?**

Well, for one thing, I'd tell them how many reported cases
there are and then I'd say, "How many people live in this
country?" and then I'd say, "What percent is that?" And say
that, while it is a problem because there's no known cure as of
yet, it's not affecting that many people. More people die in car
wrecks every day than have died from AIDS. Yet people still

drive cars. The risk is there, but to go paranoid because they think that they might have a wreck is insane to me. Also, people smoke cigarettes. They're going to die of lung cancer if they smoke cigarettes. That's why the panic with AIDS—people just need to use some common sense about it. It's bad because it has happened to so many homosexuals. I found out also that my brother was a hemophiliac.

Blood may be found to be the major, if not the only way it can be transmitted.

Right! When it comes down to it, when everything is finally known.

What is one word that summarizes your feeling about AIDS?

Anger. I just get mad as hell about the whole thing. I'm mad because my brother had it. I'm mad because he died of it. I'm mad at the public. I'm mad—I'm just mad. I'm mad because they haven't found a cure. I'm mad!

Have you evaluated your own way of living since you became aware of all this?

Not really. Long before health foods were in, we were eating fish and cutting down on red meat.

Why?

'Cause you live longer.

Where did you read that?

I didn't have to read that. I know it. I mean, putting red

meat into your body always sounded to me a little bit ridiculous. I come from a meat-and-potatoes type family. Well, I
guess that's probably where it all came from. And all of those
people always had a lot of health problems. Everybody in my
family was overweight and had a lot of health problems. If you
looked at what they ate, it was red meat, potatoes, and pasta.
So it only made sense to me when I was a kid that, hey, if I
don't eat white bread 'cause that equals white death—

(Laughs.)

I'm getting into some books now about life extension. I've
always believed that if you took good care of your body, that it
would serve you. Because like I said, I was a sick kid when I
was a kid, and I've always felt that through proper maintenance I would be healthier. But I'm a boring person.

No, don't say that. Continue what you were saying.

Well, it's just like a car. You change the oil and the spark
plugs—

Uh-huh. But why do all this? What was your motive?

Well, proper maintenance means longer life.

**I see. How did your family cope with your brother's ill-
ness?**

Well, my wife took it probably as hard as I did. She really
did. She had a lot of sympathy and compassion for my
brother. There was one cousin of mine that we both—my
brother and I—always felt more close to. I guess she's about
fifty years old now. And my brother and I talked to her and
told her what his problem was and the fact that he did have

AIDS and all. This particular cousin happens to live in the same town as my in-laws, and she knows who my in-laws are. She ran into my mother-in-law and did the whole thing with her about AIDS and Bob staying with us and our two kids and this and that. And my in-laws acted like real assholes.

We went back to my hometown and had a memorial service and all. And my in-laws live in a town about sixty miles away, so we were going to fly in and go down to the in-laws and then go over to my house. Because of geography it would have been easier to do it that way, to stay the night at her parents' house than go to my house. But when she called, she said her twin sister told us not to come. We had all four been exposed to the infection, so therefore we were all lepers. That really hurt—that really hurt my wife a lot. A lot.

Did the kids have a hard time from other people?

Just from the in-laws, because those were really the only people that knew that my brother had AIDS. In fact, I never told my Dad, 'cause I didn't want to hear it from him.

Would you describe what your brother's physical condition was? Describe what he was like physically, what you had to do for him?

His physical condition for the entire time he was here reminds me of what you see in the newsreels of the Jews in the Nazi concentration camps: just skin and bones.

Like malnutrition?

Yeah, exactly. His doctor from San Francisco said that was part of AIDS. We had a dietary supplement thing for him to drink that got all involved; and that's really about the only thing that he would take. It was forcing him to do that. He

didn't want to eat anything. He didn't even want the food sup-
plements. Unless we sat there and actually coaxed him on to
drinking it, he wouldn't.

We tried to have him at the dinner table with us to blend
him in with the family life. That didn't work. Well, it worked
for two weeks. Then it didn't work. So then I was sleeping in
the room with him and having my breakfast with him and having my dinner with him and keeping him company and all.

That was okay with the rest of the family?

I really didn't ask. (They laugh.) The kids sort of complained a little bit because we were spending so much time
with him.

Did they get close to him at all?

They always used to be.

Was he mentally alert when he was home?

For the first week or so he was. Of course, over Thanksgiving it was just "Uncle Bob," and foolin' around with Uncle
Bob, but when he came back, they saw the—the marked
change in him. And they sort of left him alone. They would
talk to him and go around him, but only if he really sort of
wanted them to. In other words, they gave him some space.

**What do you think about democracy in American govern-
ment now?**

Everybody should be left to do what they want. That's
what democracy is. (Chuckles.) I think that I hate lawyers.

Why?

Because lawyers make laws, and they make the laws so that they have a job. Things get more screwed up and more screwed up because they try to make things more intricate and more intricate. Well, that's how I feel about it.

Have your values about life and death changed in the last few months?

They really haven't. Life is here to enjoy and to make the best possible world here that you can, and death comes to us all and it's just a matter of when. I am getting sort of paranoid about driving, because a drunk driver slid into me about a month ago. I've seen about four different car wrecks since that time, and I was talking to a guy yesterday, and *he* was in a car wreck. You just never know, so why worry about it?

Life is just a stage, and after this life you go on to another life. And that is really the only spiritual belief I have. It's not really spiritual because it comes to all people. The next life is different, and this life is just practice and training for the next. This life is childhood. (Laughs.) You go to the next one, and the next life is kindergarten, then the one after that is grade school. Life is just progression.

What about religion and AIDS? Any comments about that?

Well, I think that religion is a good business to get into, because there's a lot of money to be made. As far as what other people do, they have to live with themselves, 'cause religion is all a hustle.

What do you think about mainstream medicine and AIDS?

They're doing what they can.

What about alternative medicine?

Well, that—that is probably the best way. But, to begin with, you have to find the ones that work for AIDS. Until you can find them, there's nothing you really can do. There's a lot that goes into mainstream research. Alternative-type medicine is, I think, again, probably the best, but at the same time, you have to know what you're trying to deal with to begin with. So that's where the big-time laboratories and research facilities really play the role, to tell you what you're trying to go against. I think that the government should stay out of it and let private industry take care of it.

11

Wisdom and Grace

Lu Chaikin

Lu Chaikin is a psychotherapist who lives and practices in San Francisco. She is a lesbian in her late fifties and is in generally good health, except for arthritis. Her colleague and close friend, Gary Walsh, also a psychotherapist, died of AIDS on February 21, 1984, a year and one month after being diagnosed.

I

When did you first become aware of AIDS?

It was about two years ago. It was before Gary was diagnosed, which was on January 22, 1983. It was about six months or a year before that that I began to hear about it.

Where did you first hear of it? What was the source of the knowledge?

I think probably gay newspapers. I work in the Castro; my office is there. And from clients—about half my practice is men. So we just began to hear about it in the air, kind of.

What was your first contact with a person with AIDS?

I knew of Paul Dague, and I would meet him on the street now and again.

How many people now do you know who have AIDS?

It must be about six.

What was the warning sign that really signaled to Gary that something was going haywire?

Generally, he didn't feel well, but the specific was a lesion. He had a lesion on his leg in December before he and Joe went off to Key West. Then he came back in January and went to the doctor; it was confirmed, and I will *never* forget the day he came into the office. Just one look at his face, and I knew. We went into his office—we both had clients waiting for us—and sat down and cried; we talked for a while, and then went to work.

My first reaction, hearing more and more about AIDS, was that it was a death sentence, and what I see that I did, in retrospect, was to go into mourning. The first month or two, I was depressed out of my mind and saw Gary as dead, practically. I realize now I had to go through that in order to come back to, "He has an indeterminate amount of time, but he does have *some* time, and I'm going to do my best to make that time as rich as possible." So you have to go through death to come back to life, at least in that particular way.

During that period of time, was his physical experience of the illness what you expected it would be?

I really wasn't close enough to have a great deal of expectation. He was *exhausted*. He was very, very tired for several months before the diagnosis, and I knew that that was one of the symptoms. And he had night sweats and skin disorders. But as I went through it with him—and this was daily contact; if I didn't see him, we'd be on the phone every day for an hour. After work, I would talk to him. So I went through every symptom and every pimple and every rash and pain and ache and terror and hope and the whole thing.

How about other people's reactions to him?

They varied. Some people—the good folks—were just tremendous, enormously supportive and caring, an outpouring of love and concern. There were some people who were almost indifferent; in fact, some people that he had worked with daily, he just didn't hear from. And one friend, a friend of his from New York, did deny him. He lost that friend, who couldn't take it. But that was very rare. Mostly it was the opposite; the best in people came out. That was partly who Gary was.

How do you perceive that people are at risk for getting AIDS?

Well, I don't think you have to be promiscuous, whatever that means. I think one or two contacts can do it. From everything I read—and I've read a *lot* of stuff—it does seem to be transmitted sexually. And I think that it probably is exchange of bodily fluid. My hunch is, probably most gay men in San Francisco have already been exposed, and some are going to get it and some aren't. But I think it can be one contact or a person whose system is not in good shape generally, and maybe it is associated in some people with breaking down of the body through excess drug use or antibiotics and all the rest, or constitutional weakness or whatever. I don't know.

How do you think persons with AIDS are at risk for catching other infections?

I think they're at a high risk. I do belieive that, because the immune system is down and you're a sitting duck, as it were.

How did you control against Gary's risk of catching a cold from you or something?

If I had a cold, which I don't think I did while Gary was ill, if he were in the hospital or at home, I wouldn't visit. In the hospital, they have those masks. But I was not ill during the time with Gary. In the office, I did have one cold. I think I would just try not to be very close, and cover my nose and mouth when sneezing or whatever.

What is "risky sex"?

I think probably one of the major, riskiest kinds of sex is things like fisting, because I think that breaks down the tissue. If there's semen that then enters into the anal area, which is contaminated or whatever you want to call it, somehow that seems to be the riskiest.

What is "safe sex"?

Well, "safe sex" would be where there's no exchange of bodily fluid at all, which would be mutual masturbation and other body contact, but "no fucking, no sucking." (They laugh.)
No fun, huh?

So basically you believe in these definitions of "safe" versus "risky" sex?

I think at this point I do, and I'm like a Jewish mother with some of the men clients I have about their sexual practices. You know, if in doubt, why put yourself on the lines to be shot? You know?

How do you control against catching AIDS?

I did think about it a little bit with Gary, because I'd kiss him and hug him every time we saw each other, but not on the mouth, and I ate over there a great deal. But I did once, I remember, have some funny purple spot somewhere on my body, I don't remember where, and I thought, "Oh, my God!" You know? Would I get AIDS? And I thought about that for a while, and I guess I thought it was possible. And then I asked myself, "Would I do anything differently with Gary?" and the answer was clearly no. So it may be an illusion, but I guess I think from what we know of what's going on, I probably am not at risk, so I don't think about it too much. When I do think about it, it just boggles my mind how gay men have to cope. I just think it's horrendous. And for some, I think it's a relief when they get it, because they're so worried. At least they know.

Several of my clients are physicians, and one was telling me the other day he had talked to somebody who is doing research and is "in the know" because of whatever he's doing, and he predicted that AIDS would go up to five percent of the gay male population, because it was incrementally increasing by half a percent a month or however the increments were. That would be one out of twenty. Now, that is the most pessimistic estimate that I've heard.

And that only includes the gay population. That doesn't speak to its spreading elsewhere.

Correct. Now, that was the only thing that got to him. He'd been reasonably safe before, and when he heard that, I could tell that that really got to him. He just came back from a trip to Europe, and when Americans go over there and talk "safe sex" with some of these Europeans, these Europeans just look at them like, "You're crazy." You know, "This isn't any fun." Even out of San Francisco, in smaller towns, traveling in this country, there are not the precautionary measures that are taken here.

Sure. How do you think the government should stop AIDS from spreading?

I think the main thing the government can do is financial. There are other things, such as educational; they certainly could do a great deal with that for both the gay population—or people at risk—and the general population. But I think funding, as they would do if this hit any other population—if this were hitting children, for example, or just Middle America—

More than it is.

Yes, I think they're beginning now—the latest thing I read in *B.A.R.*, as a matter of fact, yesterday, was that $93 million, which was what was asked for by the researchers, was granted. It was $40 million more than Reagan proposed, and he was against this amount. So I think actually money for research is probably the major thrust. In regard to Middle America's reaction to AIDS, in addition to anger, I feel great sadness that our countrymen and women are so callous and uncaring about the suffering of others. That they allow their prejudices to overcome their humanity. This is reflected in the government's response to the crisis as well.

How has the AIDS crisis made you feel?

I feel everything. I feel anger; I feel great sadness; I feel grateful for myself. When you are close to death, it makes you look at your own life. So the self-examination has been stimulated greatly through my contact with AIDS, and Gary in particular.

What kinds of emotions have you experienced in terms of changes in the gay community or gay identity?

In my privileged position of seeing gay men, it's been fascinating to me. The scary, the "negative" parts of this aside, I think it has helped an enormous number of men to reevaluate their own lives. Sex was used as an escape, a way to let off steam, a way to express oneself in the gay community, as you know. That was the major outlet for a lot of emotions: the need for connection, anger, wanting closeness—physical closeness would do if they couldn't make an emotional contact.

I've found that when the sexual avenue is diminished—cut off or diminished—and some men have been celibate for a year or two, that I've known—it opens up other avenues. And so men have begun to see other men as people, and there have been other ways to relate. They've been forced to find other ways to relate to other men as well as finding other ways to express themselves. And that has been, to a large extent, quite enriching.

I think also, in a way, it's pulled the gay community together. It's opened a great deal of compassion and support for one another. This dreadful epidemic has facilitated the maturing of the gay male community. Its sobering effect has resulted in more cohesiveness, more caring, and more genuine emotional expression toward one another. It's as though the community were in its adolescence before and is now painfully entering manhood.

In terms of your emotional experiences, how has society's reaction to AIDS made you feel?

Well, I guess it makes me angry that people treat people with AIDS as lepers. And it's a sad commentary that our country—you know, it's almost like they refuse to be informed.

And it just—I don't know, it's very frustrating. It does not make me feel proud to be an American, if this is the way people—I'm sure it's not just a national phenomenon. But mostly it makes me—it upsets me a lot.

II

In the obituary in the *Bay Area Reporter* you shared the one thing that Gary had given you was to teach you about love. Would you care to describe what you meant by that?

Yes, I'd be glad to. Gary was one of the most loving people I've ever met. I feel that our relationship provided me with the experience closest to unconditional love that I'll probably ever have in my life. And he was a very compassionate man as well, and very sensitive, and exceedingly intuitive, so that knowing him was a gift. I mean, it really was a gift. He was an extraordinary man and an exceptionally fine therapist because of his qualities.

With Gary, I felt more ability to be myself and to be vulnerable and to be loving than I ever have. And, as a consequence, close as we were when he was diagnosed, the closeness increased exponentially during the year and month after his diagnosis. We just opened up and opened up and opened up to each other. It was like we touched souls, literally. I know it's a hackneyed phrase.

And I could see also how he affected other people, because I was there a lot when people would visit. By being himself, he brought out the soft side in people who would ordinarily just not let that out. So, he just *was* love, you know? And by being who he was—and he moved into that more and more—he was transformed and he transformed other people.

And there's a kind of depth that he had and he just touched people in ways which would enable them to not only experience the softer, tenderer side of themselves, but enabled them to look at themselves somehow and grow through contact with him. And it's hard to believe the letters and the phone calls and the responses that people had to him.

There was a videotape of him—I don't know if you have time to see it—that Shanti has. In fact, I have a copy, too. He talks about working in New York in a tough neighborhood and being a social worker there and working with these tough cookies and crazies and everything else, and he said, "I'd always go for the heart." And he said, "I just would always make a connection when I went for the heart." And that's what he did.

And I find that whatever I've been going through, which is very enormous, through the experience with Gary and since he's died, has enabled me to expand and incorporate my own version of the Gary that I love more than I ever have before. You know, my own ability to be compassionate and caring and more tender.

Could you describe the stages you went through from Gary's diagnosis to his death to now?

As I did say earlier, in the beginning, I reacted as though he were dead, practically. And then came "Round Two: He isn't dead," and living every moment much more fully with him. I mean, every moment was precious. We had visits and conversations and contacts that were so—I don't know. I don't know how to describe it. They were just so wonderful and loving and caring and—it was just marvelous. There are no words for the kind of experience we had together. It was exceedingly close. Underlying the time after I came from—mentally—his dying, of course, was the notion that he probably would die, which made every moment richer.

There was another layer of his health, because for a while he didn't feel too bad. Then, after pneumocystis, he was feeling dreadful, and it was one thing after another. He was in a *lot* of pain and great fatigue. He just had a limited amount of time. There were some periods when he was up and out of bed maybe six or seven hours a day and that was it, and just be around his apartment. So that time for me was a time of giving to my fullest, which enabled me, of course, to receive very, very fully.

And he had two months in December and January—it was like a Christmas gift, you know—where he felt a lot better. He even was out shopping for Christmas things. And we had spent Thanksgiving together, he and Matthew and another friend and myself, and also Christmas and New Year's. The three of us—Matthew, Gary, and I—went to see *Dream Girls*. (Laughs.) And it was a *wonderful* evening. So there was a little respite of two months where he was feeling a lot better; and there was a moment of hope in that time, you know, always tinged with telling myself, "Now, don't go overboard, and don't be foolish, and blah-blah-blah," but there was hope.

And then in February he took a turn for the worse and went into the hospital. Ironically, he was getting his apartment together and he had gone out shopping for a few end tables and this and that. I guess Matthew and I were there when Gary went to the hospital, the last time we took him, and as he was leaving his apartment, his new furniture to complete the apartment was arriving, literally. I mean, it was like passing in the doorway, and he never got back to the apartment.

So, he was in the hospital about three weeks and it was fairly clear that he would not—in the beginning it wasn't. It was one of the minor things, but after a week or so it was fairly clear that he was deteriorating fast. And I was beginning to—I felt myself kind of like pulling myself together for the end. It was not my time to fall apart; I just had to wait for that. And he asked me to be with him when he talked to the doctor when he told him that he no longer wanted any heroic measures or anything aside from just sustaining him, no remedial measures of any kind. And he wanted me to be there so his doctor would take him seriously, and also just for his own strength. And I was, and that, of course, was truly the beginning of the end.

I must say that all of us—he, Matthew, and I—the humor was there till the last minute. There was an enormous amount of humor. One night in the hospital when we were planning Gary's memorial service, we were roaring with laughter at some of the wild and crazy things that we came out with. It's hard to describe, you know, but it was sustaining in some ways.

Was it nervous laughter?

No, it was just—for example, occasionally he'd talk about suicide, and we were sitting there talking and he said, "Well, the thing about it"—and he knew that to commit suicide, you take these pills and those pills and drink alcohol with it because that makes the pills act more effectively—so he said, "Well, I've thought about suicide and taking all those pills and drinking brandy, but it worries me that they'll smell alcohol on my breath." So there was a long pause, and finally I said, "Well, ah, Gary, there won't be any breath." And he said, "Oh! Thank God! I've been worrying about that for days!" And we were hysterical; we were just hysterical. I mean, it was crazy humor.

He was in a coma, practically, the last days, and he came out of the coma and I did something or said something when he looked at me, and he said, "You are a smart cookie," you know, and "cookie" is the term I always use and he, then, began to use it, too.

He died on February twenty-first. It was a Tuesday morning.

Where were you?

I was there. It was Sunday when the last of friends and relatives left, and I turned to Matthew and I said, "Matthew, I'm not leaving." And he looked at me, because he knows I'm one for creature comfort and my own bed. I said, "I'm just *not* leaving." And, fortunately, that time was the only time he was in a room with another bed. It was a double room, but he was the only patient in it. And so I figured I'd just sleep in the other bed, and Matthew decided to stay also, so they put a cot there. And I had been worried that I wouldn't know what to do when, you know, when would I know when to cancel this and do that? But it was so clear to me. It was just so clear to me.

How?

I just knew intuitively that I could not leave and would not leave. I mean, they could not have thrown me out of that hospital. And I told Gary, and he said, "It's not going to be a picnic, you know. It's not like having a pajama party." I said, "I know that." And the first night that both of us stayed *was* horrible. He was coughing and he was having trouble breathing and the nurse was in and out and all that stuff; I think I got three hours' sleep. He was on morphine drip by then. So I just stayed.

There's one thing I do want to tell you, which I think was the most moving moment of my life. That Sunday, Joe was the last person to see him, of friends and relatives. Clearly, Matthew and I were "family" and there was not going to be a good-bye scene; we would just be there. Joe left, and I had always seen the effect that Gary had on other people, and Gary never could see it. You know, and he would say, "He feels awkward; he feels this; he feels that," and he never really honored that spectacular influence he had on other people.

So after Joe left and Matthew and Joe were talking, I walked into Gary's room and somehow I just wanted him to know that; he had to know that. So I said to him, "Gary, you just have to know the effect you have on other people." I said, "I just saw Joe"—and we had talked about this quite a bit— and finally he said, "I know." He said, "I finally got it." And he said, "I *am* love and light, and I transform people by just being who I am." Whereupon I wept, I just cried, and we held each other.

And there was a little brass statue of a magician that Jim Geary had given him for Christmas, and I adored it; I just thought it was wonderful. And he had it in the hospital, and he reached over to his side table and he said, "I want to give this to you while I'm still alive." And it was like the passing of a baton or something, you know? And it's my most cherished possession. And so he finally did get it, and I felt so good and it was like a completion for us.

Sunday was a very hard day for everybody, Gary in particular. And Monday, he went into a coma, I guess in early evening, and then Tuesday morning, he died. And even then, he waited until Matthew and I woke up and had a little breakfast, and he was in a coma.

There was one time, Matthew and I were on the side of the bed, one on each side, holding Gary's hands. He was in a semicoma, and we were talking to him, how much we loved him, and how much we got from him, and it's okay to let go, and all of this, and just back and forth, Matthew would talk and I would talk. I guess we weren't holding his hand, we were holding his arm, and he had his hands in front of him on his chest. And a little technique I learned from hypnosis—because he couldn't respond; he was, as I say, kind of in a semi-coma—I touched his index finger, and I said, "Gary, if you can hear us, just move your finger as much as you can." And there was no response, and I did it again: "If you can hear us, move your finger." And then his finger just moved a little bit, and so we knew we were still making contact, and of course, Matthew's eyes bugged out and his mouth opened. And so we just continued to keep up that contact because we knew that he was hearing us. And so we would do that periodically through the day, and then there was a point when he went into a very deep coma and clearly I don't think we were reaching him anymore.

Could you sense a departing from him?

Yes and no. I was so zonked and exhausted and had taken, I don't know what, some of his pills to go to sleep, which didn't work, so I was just kind of spacey, but I guess that morning, I just knew. I had had other experiences of closeness with him, but that does not answer your question. I knew he was going, but I didn't know that that minute would be the departure of the spirit or that sort of thing.

Had you been with anyone before when they had passed?

No. The closest was when my father died. My parents were living in San Mateo and my mother called me and I went down, and it was a half hour after he died, but not at the moment of departure.

It was so interesting to me, I came home—and I had, for purposes of convenience, declared myself his aunt, since I'm nineteen years older than he, for papers and hospital stuff and all that junk, so it would expedite the procedure. So after all of that was done, several hours after he died, I came home, and I stepped in the front door and the first thing I wanted to do was to go to the phone and call Gary and tell him what happened.

I always called Gary, no matter what happened! If it was of any consequence at all. And I stood there like I was in shock. That's when it really hit me. I couldn't call Gary anymore! And the loss, the emptiness, the void was tremendous! (Crying.) I mean, I knew—I knew there'd be a gaping hole inside of me, but that was the first glimmer I had of it.

He knew this, before he passed, that he would leave behind people who would hurt?

Yes, and in the tape, he talks about that. That hurt him most. He just was so unhappy about that and he just felt so bad and so sad, mostly for Matthew and me, and others, that his departure would cause us pain.

Yet he spoke of death as a relief and a joy, at times.

He did. He went through everything. You know, there were times he was terrified, times he looked upon it as an exciting adventure, something he hadn't done before, and other times the great sense of peace and equanimity and relief—you know, relief from the fatigue and the pain.

I had not realized how much pain was involved in this disease. I had not realized it. Nobody told me, and Gary didn't, either. It was an enormous amount of terrible pain: awful headaches, bone aches, muscle aches, aside from the sweats and other things. So it was a relief.

I do want to tell you what I'm going through now, because for months—the first few months were so awful, I can't tell you. You know, the sense of loss and the grief and despair and—you know. I knew I would get through it, but the getting through it was dreadful, and I also let myself be as open as I possibly could to everything I had to feel. So I didn't see a lot of people very much. I just wanted—I *needed* a lot of time to myself. So it was just people like Matthew and other really close friends that I saw, and after two weeks I went back to work. Work is always therapeutic for me, and I'm much better at my work than at home. (Laughs.)

But about a month ago, I had to clean out that little room over there, and I have Gary's journals, and I have been assiduously avoiding them because I knew I just couldn't take it. I was in that room and there was this bag full of Gary's journals, and I just sat down and started reading them. I was all prepared to be devastated, and it was very interesting, what happened. I wasn't devastated. In fact, it was like a wonderful visit with him.

None of what he wrote was surprising, and he wrote a *lot* about his relationship with Matthew and falling in love with Matthew and their relationship and separating from Matthew (laughs) and all of that stuff. And then when he was diagnosed and not feeling well, he was much less people and much more internal, all of which—really, all of which—we had talked about.

But the odd thing that happened was that somehow I realized I had deified him, and I could allow him, after reading the journals, for some reason, to be a person. And what happened was that the heaviness that I had been carrying around for seven months or so dissipated, and I felt—though I had been feeling it for a year and certainly the six months since Gary died—I felt an opening in myself take what was like a quantum leap. I took on more of the characteristics that I talked about before: my own accessibility to my own loving, caring feelings and compassion. They were also there, you know; we all have them, but they had been opening more and more, and slowly, and it was like a big jump, and I just *felt* softer and more tender and more open.

You had received his gift.

That's right. Yes, it was a stimulation of who I was, but I let him hold it, for the most part, those qualities, as he let me hold the more assertive. We talked about this at great length, because I was more assertive and more willing to stick my neck out about certain things. We realized that in our relationship I taught him how to be more of a man and he taught me how to be more of a woman. We had each developed the other side more because of our own experiences. All along we were open with each other and talked about this stuff and realized, as unlikely a pair as we seemed, the depth of the connection and what we were learning from each other. We often commented on the fact that we were each other's best teacher, aside from our own internal teaching.

You referred to him as though he were a hero, in a sense, and the heartbreak evolved in some way to make him not so much a hero, but—

I'm not exactly sure, but more human and, I think, allowing myself to expand and take on some of those characteristics allowed me to sort of let go of the acute grief. I mean, I still have a grief, but not the acute grief. I'm not there yet; I feel as though I'm right in the middle of this process—the acute grieving, the moving into the less acute but still there, and I know in my heart that there's a way to connect with Gary that's not through sadness. (Crying.) I know there's a way for me to connect with him through the joy that we experienced, and I don't know how I'm going to get there, but I just know that that's the next place to go.

I think Gary's capacity for his emotional experience was huge; it was enormous. And mine was, too, but it was skewed differently. And we connected on a basic level and then taught ourselves—taught each other. We taught ourselves, too, using the other as a model, in a sense, filling out our own self.

In fact, upon his death, there was an absorption, if you will; there's something that remains with you. And there is this—I've heard this proposed—kind of a notion that some people are sacrifices for others. And, putting it in that context, Gary's contribution was extraordinarily and dramatically heightened because he died; his contribution to other people.

What was his contribution to other people?

His contribution was that deeply accepting and loving quality that he had that made room for people to move, to grow and expand. That he was so accepting and also intuitive and could also tell you—you know, sometimes I'd call him up and not know what was going on in my own head. I didn't know what I felt until I talked to him, and then he'd tell me. (Laughs.) You know, then we'd talk about it and I'd know.

So it was that great compassion and acceptance, coupled with being a loving person, that allowed people to move out of themselves, to move and to expand their own experience. That often happens in therapy, but that's how he lived. But he had these qualities to such great measure that the daily contact with him, or *any* contact with him, was a privilege. I mean, it really was.

And people would call and leave messages on his machine, and they'd want to see him for ten minutes or this and that. Of course, when his energy level was low, he just couldn't. And he learned, hard as it was for him, to say no to people. He learned how to take care of himself, finally, because he had to.

III

Gary Walsh was on a television special where he spoke with Reverend Jerry Falwell. Can you describe what that was about?

Oh, this was my least favorite TV exposure, because Falwell is so aggravating. Falwell was doing his usual trip of quoting the Bible and saying homosexuality is a sin, but he loves homosexuals; you know, that kind of "crapola." And of course it wasn't just Gary; there were several other panelists. The thing that stands out in my mind is that people would talk on this intellectual level and Gary cut through that shit so beautifully.

First of all, Falwell would say, *"Gary,* this and that." Gary came back with, "Well, *Jerry,"* which I adored. Because we had often talked, and I have this thing about doctors who call you by your first name, and here I am, twice as old, maybe, as some of these guys. So they say, "Well, Lu." I say right away, "Well, Dick, how I feel is," or whatever, you know. So he was saying, "Well, Jerry."

Jerry was saying at one point, "I really love you," you know, sort of, even though we were homosexual. And Gary said, "You know, I'm not insensitive, but I don't feel any love coming from you at all." And it was *the* sentence in the whole program that cut through the crap, and it was incredible. And Falwell didn't know what to say, and so he was flustered a moment and then started shoveling shit again.

What was Gary's reaction after the television program? What did he go through?

Matthew was actually at the television station. Gary had mixed feelings: "Oh, I should have said this, I should have said that," and also feeling good about other things. He was quite nervous beforehand, of course. But he felt good about *that* part, you know, because that's where Gary was at his best, getting right into the feelings. He invited Falwell to come to San Francisco, and of course Falwell said a general, "Oh, yeah." I thought it was really not a debate, like the presidential debates; it was a hoopla thing.

How did Gary deal with the question of "Why me?"

I think at first there was some "Why me?" and anger and pain about that, but I think eventually he saw it in the greater scheme of things, like "it had to be him." His last year, he wrote in his journal—and we had talked about it as well—he said, "There are so many wonderful things happening to me now." He said, "I wouldn't miss any of it." There were times he got to a place where he realized he never could have the experience he was having unless he were in this situation, dying and everybody knowing it, including himself.

Did he go through different stages of adjusting?

Oh, yes, I think, yes. I think the first was kind of shock and horror and disbelief and also some relief at just being able to tell all his clients. One week, he told all his clients, and it was a complete turnaround. Here's the healer, saying "I'm sick," and the client really moving in—and this was another funny thing, you know—tearful sessions with clients, and we would joke about the clients coming out of his office with all these tears, and my clients thinking, "God, they probably had a great session!" (Laughs.)

I said, "Gary, you're killing my business!" So here's the kind of humor that we had all along. You know, we'd laugh, and the underlying tragedy was always there. So there was that stage, and I think numbness. Probably a person who's dying goes through all the grieving stages that the people who are left behind go through, and everyone does it at his or her pace.

When did you first see that he was beginning to grieve?

Well, I knew he was disturbed and worried before he was diagnosed. And I think he went into some kind of mourning period after the diagnosis.

When did the phase of sort of seeing death as a relief come?

It would vary. He would have some of these wonderful moments—by moments, you know, it could be days or whatever—and then some other thing would happen. Either he'd get another infection or for some reason or another he became depressed—he had a lot of reasons to be depressed—and he knew he had to go into himself. And frequently he would just do that, and maybe not even talk to me that day, and just say, "I just have to be by myself." And he would go into himself and sit with himself and be depressed and deal witih it, live through it.

And then he would always come out on a different level. And he knew that was his process, and he hated it because it was so painful, and he could tell it was coming. But that's what he would do. He never avoided it; he would always go into it and go with it. And that was his great strength: He just never went around this stuff or tried to avoid it; he went into it. And I learned a lot from that.

It sounds like you and Matthew were his closest support. What other kinds of support did he have?

He had other friends and also he did go to a Shanti group.

What did he perceive as support, and what could he not tolerate any longer from people?

Well, clearly, he could not tolerate phoniness. I've talked about his well-developed intuition a number of times, and he just knew what people felt and how they felt. He would tell me sometimes that he would be on the street and see somebody and they would say, "How *are* you?" And he would want to throw up. He'd say, *"Fine!* How are *you?"* You know, just that kind of maudlin sort of approach, that phony caring. He really did sort out the trivia and the insincere, and he just knew. And what support for him was, was a genuineness in somebody, and he didn't want to be protected.

Let me tell you one incident which is so typically Gary. While he was still up and about, we would sometimes meet for lunch, and one day we met for lunch on Castro and he had just been to the doctor's and was talking about that and what the doctor said, and then he said to me, "How do *you* feel? I mean, how are *you* dealing with all this?" And I was just so overwhelmed by that question because, somehow, here he was, he was the patient, he had just come from the doctor, he'd just had bad news, and he was asking me how I was. And it just touched me so deeply, and I told him. And he said, "I don't want you not to tell me how you feel." He said, "I want to know." And we made an agreement then that we would not protect each other, that we would talk to each other, you know, continue to talk to each other from our hearts.

I told him how difficult it was for me, and one of the early things that struck me when he was diagnosed was that he wasn't going to be there for me when I died. (Her voice breaks.) That was the way it was supposed to be, and he wasn't going to be there. And that just upset me so much, in addition to just contemplating the loss of Gary in my life. And I had sort of a vision after he died, and I knew that he would be there. I mean, it was like I saw him, and it was typically like across a line or a little river or something. I saw myself dying, and I saw Gary standing there, helping me across, and being there for me. And he often said, "You're not going to be able to get rid of me as easily as you think!" (Laughs.) He said, "I'm going to be there." And I saw then how, in one of the many ways, he would be there for me when I die.

You mentioned earlier that you had changed, that you'd gone through some self-evaluations.

Well, one of the big things is how I spend my time. Time is so much more precious to me. The dying truly do teach the living about life, I think. And I'm more congruent. I mean, I don't do many things I don't want to do. There are always a few, I think, in life, and there are just some things you just have to do. But it's a minimum. So that's a major thing in terms of doing what I want to do with my time. It is my time, and time is the only irreplaceable thing that we have.

I was never a big bullshitter, but I'm less so now. You know, I really am much more open, I think, as a result of this experience with Gary. I've also thought a lot more about my own finiteness and my own death. It was sort of coming slowly anyway; it does with age. I think fifty was a big year for me in terms of truly realizing that I wasn't going to be here forever.

But this has changed your values about life and death, or about mortality?

Well, when I talk about my own finiteness, it makes me realize—you know how people are; they don't think of their own deaths. You know, it's hard to conceive of your own death. But I'm getting closer to that, realizing that I really will die. The statistics are ten out of ten, right? And it's gotten me on a whole trip about death and what is that all about, and what do I believe? I'm not really sure. I'm not really sure that the spirit lives on. I like to think so, and sometimes I feel that that's probably so. That's all kind of in flux for me. But it's much more present, and it makes time more precious as well.

How did Gary value death? What were his attitudes about death and the spirit and the hereafter?

He felt that there definitely was a spiritual life after death, and in some ways, some odd things happened. For example, here it is, eight months after Gary's death, and last week I was talking to Matthew and we both said to each other how much we had been thinking of Gary that day. That was a week ago Friday, and I don't think that's accidental. So funny little things happen, but he did truly feel that his spirit would live on. He didn't know in what form. I remember, we were talking about that in the hospital and he had a very mischievious look in his eye, and I said, "You're really curious about this. You're excited about this, aren't you?" And he said, "Yeah." So there was that—a new place to explore.

Well, it is an exploration and it is a new horizon. Right after Gary's diagnosis, maybe two months after the diagnosis, did he go through a period of sort of taking stock?

I'm sure he did. I think in the beginning he thought he would go back to work, so he didn't think he was done. He was planning on, well in two months, and three months, and so forth, that he would go back to work. I don't remember that as being a major topic. I'm sure he did, himself, and I think the culminating thing to whatever stock he was taking was that incident I told you of, in the hospital, when he realized that he did transform people's lives by being who he was, and that he was love and light. So that had to be the end of a long process that he had been going through. I'm sure there are things I've forgotten. I probably should have kept a journal, but I didn't.

Did he feel singled out for misfortune or that he had done something to deserve this?

A little; he said the Catholic church kind of snuck in there every now and again, and he did go through periods of "It's because I'm gay, and God's punishing me." And his parents, of course, were no help at all. His mother wanted him to go back to the holy church and all that stuff. He did get to the point where he could always know whether to knock it off, if the conversations were either going to be decent or not at all, and he didn't want to hear all that crap. I mean, he said it nicely, but he said it. They never did come out, and he never asked them to come out. They live in Iowa.

Were they accepting of his homosexuality before?

No; didn't speak to him for three years. And that was just kind of getting together a little bit, and then he was diagnosed.

IV

Have your beliefs about gay freedom changed any as a result of AIDS?

Interesting question. I don't know that they've changed

basically. I think I was a pretty strong proponent of people doing what they need to or want to do, as long as it isn't harmful to anybody, and I think homosexuality certainly fits in that category. I think that somehow this plague is solidifying the gay community. But my views have not really changed.

How about your views of American democracy?

(Laughs.) You certainly do ask simple questions! I've been a cynic from way back, so this doesn't change things a lot for me. I had maybe twenty or thirty years ago realized that when you think about the rise and fall of a civilization, I have felt Western democracy is in a decline. I haven't seen anything in the last twenty years to indicate that something's happening to the contrary. Maybe if I were twenty-five years old, my answers would be different to those questions, but I was pretty well formulated by last year, so things haven't changed that much in the global picture.

In general, what would you say about how the biological family has responded?

For the most part, in my experience and people that I have known, most families have rallied and really come through. There are some who haven't. There are the horror stories, but most families, I think, have come through quite well.

Does it change the family?

Oh, I think it brings them closer. It definitely brings them closer, and allows them to communicate in a way they never had before. In fact, one of my clients, who was diagnosed just a few days prior to my seeing him, was going back to the Midwest to tell his family number one, that he was gay, number two, that he has AIDS. And I'm sure—I just have a sense that if it does anything at all good, it brings them closer.

How about mainstream medicine? How do you think it defines and treats individuals and the symptoms of AIDS?

I do think they're trying. I do think they are. I think they're doing what they can. I think physicians themselves are very frustrated, those that I've spoken to, you know. Their business is getting people well and here they see these young men, and many of them are gay physicians and it's kind of a double whammy. They can't make them better and they're scared for themselves. But I'm not down on mainstream medicine. I think there's room for everybody, and I think they offer, sometimes, relief, and they certainly offer relief from pain.

How do you perceive the relationship between mainstream medicine and government control?

I'm not sure. You know, I think government does control, certainly research projects, and more and more the practice of medicine, and the intrusion and payment schemes and this, that, and the other thing. But I'm not sure how to answer that question.

Well, maybe I could ask it differently. What do you think would be an effective relationship between medicine and society?

I think it should be a cooperative relationship. I think there is that "holier than thou" medical self-perception, which I think is breaking down a little bit. So I think openness on the part of medical people is very important.

What would you say an effective relationship would be

between government and medicine? For example, with the discovery of a virus by medicine, how could government respond?

I think government should be supportive; I don't think they should be meddling. If they want to do research, I think, "Here's $10 million, buddy, go to it." And then if something comes out of that research, then government should be there to facilitate the production of whatever support systems are needed in order to help the outgrowth of the research, to help with production of vaccines or whatever. But I think government should stay out of the medical business and be supportive in terms of money and facilities and systems—you know, whatever they can offer.

What about homeopathic medicine? Do you think that it offers any genuine alternatives to treatment for AIDS?

I don't know. I don't know so far that anything has been effective, homeopathic or conventional. I think homeopathic, in many instances, is probably as effective as conventional medicine for those who really can get into it. However, the outlook is bleak. So I think it probably is up to the individual to decide what suits him best and then do it, even if it's a combination of both.

But I think there's room for all of it, and I think that what homeopathic medicine offers that the other doesn't is that the person with AIDS feels as though they're much more in charge of what's going on. I think there's a benefit in terms of one's own well-being in being in charge of his life and having some feeling of control over his life. I think it may affect the course of the disease, maybe not ultimately, but I think the course of it, and also the state of mind of the patient.

Everything, I think, is psychosomatic. We have a mind

and we have a body, and they work together when things are going well. And I think if you just give up your mind and say to a doctor, "Here's my body; do something," you've cut off half your own resources. So that if you can incorporate and do both and take this emotional/psychological charge of yourself and also feel you're influencing what your body does, then I think that helps your general state of mind, perception about self, and then, consequently, where you are in the world.

If this kind of (as it's called in our field) mind/body dualism has the power to affect the course of the illness, then could it not also affect the predisposition to the illness?

It might. I think one needs more research on that, but I think it well might. I don't know where the line is; I do think there are "miracles." I think there are people with cancer, for example, who otherwise would have died, who have not died because of the way they have used their own resources and their perception and imagery and all of that. There may be some people who have survived and we don't know about them. So I think it could affect it. I don't know how you prove it or how you do it or anything, but I believe you *can* affect your body; you can do it before, during, and after a disease.

What is your perception of psychologists and the way they have dealt with this illness?

Let's see, I talked to Joe. He at one time had six clients with AIDS, and he himself has been in the hospital. I don't know, I'm off the top of my head now, but I think to the extent that the psychotherapist him- or herself is together about their perception of life and death and life-threatening illness and everything else, to that extent they would be good with AIDS clients. I think it's another sort of thing to deal with in a client, and it's not separate, so it reflects who the therapist is in terms of the work that he or she does.

So if you're asking me if good work is being done, I have this terrible "Chaikin's ten percent law," which says that only ten percent of any profession is any good, and sometimes I think I'm being generous. That goes for doctors, dentists, therapists, street sweepers, or anything else.

Well, what about volunteer counselors and volunteer groups?

I think they do an excellent job, considering that they take people with interest, which is extremely important, but not necessarily very much training. They have intensive two-weekend training and support groups for the volunteers. I think, given who they're working with, they do very well, and I think it also speaks to the real interest and desire to contribute from the volunteers' own reasons. I think, on the whole, they do very, very well.

It's interesting because I have several clients who are volunteer counselors, and I love working with them; I really do. And the ones that I've met have really been quite good, surprisingly good, and they're very much involved in their work and getting a lot out of it and doing good work.

What about women, and the way women have been involved with AIDS? Do they bring anything special to the support of people with AIDS?

Well, my bias is women bring something special to whatever they do, if they keep in touch with their womanhood, you know, not like some women in public life who have denied that. I think women of my acquaintance vary a great deal, because a lot of the women that I know don't have very many men friends. Some do, and when they do, I think they bring a kind of a womanliness, a softness, a caring that men are less able to demonstrate.

Emotional expressiveness.

Very good. Yes. They do; yes. And I think that, among men, gay men can do that better than straight men, for example, and I think women come by it much more naturally so that they can, I think, offer support in a very caring way.

And maybe make it easier to be vulnerable and to need?

Yes, yes; I see that in my own practice, where I have men who would not go to a male therapist. They purposely—and beginning unknowingly, you know; it's not a conscious thing, but it comes out that that's why they're there; and some quite consciously.

What about reactions on the part of gay men who do not have AIDS to gay men who do have AIDS? What is an effective response? You mentioned being genuine and, you know, cutting the bullshit as part of that. In general, do you have any tips for gay men in dealing with their brothers who have AIDS?

I think to be honest and open, and I think there are times, you know, like Matthew would go over there and he would say, "Well, I'm paranoid today; I have to rewash the dishes before I'll eat from them." And Gary could understand that. So to be supportive and even talk about their own fears, because if you don't, then they exist in the relationship, but they're not stated, and the person with AIDS knows it. It's there and it acts as a barrier at a time when openness is more needed than ever.

What is an effective response on the part of the gay community to public health laws that regulate sexual behavior— the bathhouse closure, for example?

When the bathhouse issue first came up, I think there was a great brouhaha about it, and everybody had an opinion— everybody. And now that it's actually been done, I hardly hear about it. It's an extraordinary thing. I think that's partly because the quality of what went on at the baths has changed so much, from wild sex to much more subdued sex, and people just haven't talked about it very much.

Personally, I opposed it on the grounds of civil rights, and I think that there are a lot of other institutions that could be— should be—monitored and closed. If you're going to do one, do them all, and I think it is discrimination, and that bothers me.

Are there any effective coping mechanisms that you think the gay community can embrace during this time, as a community?

Using their political clout, I think. And I think we are trying to do that to get what is needed in terms of research monies and facilities, housing facilities, and all the rest that AIDS people need and that the worried well need. And provide emotional support or groups or whatever—I haven't thought that through—but, in some way, provide for either meetings or rap groups or whatever to deal with concerns and fears and joys, and sharing with whatever.

How do you think AIDS is going to change coming out for future gay people?

I don't know. That's a tough one to answer. I think if

you're gay, you're gay. There may be some young men—I
think very much in a minority—who would deny their own
sexuality, who otherwise might not. I'm not sure it will affect
coming out very much, and of all the segments of gay male
society, I think the young gay men are the ones who feel the
most cheated. And some of them are living like there is no
tomorrow anyway because of that, and that may prove to be
true. But I'm not sure that it would affect coming out an awful
lot.

**What do you think is the political advantage of the AIDS
epidemic for the Christian Right?**

Well, clearly, they've been using it as "This is God's punishment for immoral and sinful behavior," and I think they'll
push it to the hilt. Aside from the obvious, I'm not sure I have
anything more to add to that.

**What do you think about the possibility of AIDS being a
genetically engineered virus that was introduced into the community by the Christian Right or the C.I.A.?**

I've heard that a lot. For a while it was very fashionable. I
can't believe it. I can't believe it; not that they wouldn't do it—
please understand—but I can't believe that they would have
the sophistication to introduce something that would affect
only one segment of the community to such an extent—sev-
enty-two percent—and not have it spread. So on that grounds
more than any other, I don't give much credence to that notion.

How do you think it's affected the lesbian community?

Well, it depends on the extent of their involvement. I

think it's affected the gay community, including lesbians, over-all in ways of maybe more cohesiveness and support and that sort of thing, but I think lesbians are affected mostly to the extent that they have gay men friends. At the Jewish gay syn-agogue, the women have given blood because there's less like-lihood that it will be contaminated. They have an ongoing blood drive, and other lesbian organizations have done other things.

Is there a resentment on the part of lesbians for gay men bringing this plague upon the gay movement?

I have read some statements to that effect from some les-bians, but I don't know anybody personally who feels that way or who's ever expressed that.

Linda Maxey, when she was speaking of Gary, said that it takes wisdom and grace to know when to get off the bat-tlefield.

Yeah.

What do you think about that statement?

I think it's wonderful. I think she's right, because it's like there's some feeling of guilt in giving up, and that's what she was talking about. It's a beautiful statement. It's quite right.

Is there anything that you would like to see recorded for history about this period of time that we have gone through and the emotional things that we've experienced?

That we came through it with wisdom and grace, that we gave the best we could in fighting this and in caring for each other, and grew in the process, individually and as a commu-nity.

12

Putting Sex in Its Place

Armistead Maupin

Armistead Maupin is a writer living in San Francisco. His collection of Tales of the City *now includes four books. The latest,* Babycakes, *was recently released by Harper and Row.*

When did you first hear about Acquired Immune Deficiency Syndrome?

When a friend of mine came down with pneumocystis in the spring of '82. Another friend rushed up weeping with a copy of *New York* magazine and said, "This is what he's got." The article was entitled "The Gay Plague" and it was so hysterical that pretty soon we were hysterical ourselves. I've read a lot more since then, of course; most of it tends to be stuff you've already heard from the personal experience of your friends.

How many people do you know who have AIDS?

Four or five, I guess. At this point.

And how close to these people are you?

One of them was essentially the person who brought me

out, the first person who made me feel good about being gay. I met him twelve years ago in Charleston, South Carolina, and over the years we've become, you know, wonderful close soulmates of a sort, recognizing our differences. He's an actor who lives in another city, but I've always thought of him as someone I would know all my life—it's that kind of a friendship.

How old is he?

He's forty-four, I guess.

What do you see happening to people with AIDS? Without using the word *AIDS*, how would you describe this illness?

The physical manifestations of it are not immediately visible, for starters. So there's no way to describe it, because I don't know how it feels myself. I can only make observations about what I imagine these people have been going through in terms of their treatment by the rest of society.

If there's any wild generalization I can make about AIDS, it's that I tend to see amongst people who have it a much more placid and reasonable reaction to the disease than I see amongst the people who don't have it. They've been relieved of that uncertainty. The bullshit has been stripped away. The so-called "worried well" are in hysterical little bitch-fights with one another.

I can't pick up a local gay paper without getting supremely depressed—not about the AIDS statistics but because gay men have been reduced to horrid little infighting sessions, blaming each other for screwing up the AIDS Foundation or selling somebody-or-other down the river. We don't have any answers right now, so people are looking for scapegoats, and because they don't think they can blame it on the straight community (whatever *that* is), they turn on each other. It's very sad.

How do you perceive your own risk for getting AIDS?

No greater or lesser than anybody else's. Well . . . that's not exactly true. To some degree, I think I may have less risk. Because many of the things being touted as safe sex now are what I like to do anyway. I tend to be a very visual person; I've always enjoyed jerking off with someone—I get immense pleasure from that. Titwork—tactile things—I can be kissing somebody while I'm jerking off, and it's as good as any intercourse.

So have you really done anything else to control your risk right now?

Sure. I don't go to the baths anymore. I've gone to the glory holes three times in the last year, and one of those times I had oral sex with someone, but most of the time I end up in a booth with a video machine.

When you're in the company of your friends who have AIDS, how do you control against contracting it?

I don't take any special measures. I have to accept that it's a question of intimate sexual contact. If I didn't, I'd go crazy, living where I live. I'm in a completely gay neighborhood—I eat breakfast at the Welcome Home—I like to be around gay people.

In terms of your own emotional experience around AIDS, how has it made you feel?

Well, it's made me less sexual, for one thing. I've always had a certain vision of homosexuality that reaches beyond the sexual aspect of it; I can go without having sex for a long time and still feel gay as can be. I wish that more gay people would learn to do that, to feel that wonderful sense of community without needing the sex to reinforce it. I think that's a function of my age and experience as much as anything else. When I first started coming out in the early '70s, I remember how very important it was for me to go out four or five times a week and find another man. I don't devalue that experience at all; I just don't need it anymore. I find it less than satisfying.

Has AIDS changed your notion of coming out homosexual?

No. Not a bit. I do, however, think that some gay men have allowed the crisis to reinforce their latent homophobia.

When you use the word *homophobia*, what do you mean?

Just a hatred of their own sexuality. Lacking a full acceptance of who and what they are and their right to be who and what they are.

Has this changed your own needs for emotional intimacy? Or your relationships with other men?

I don't think so. Actually, my current sexual restraint has made it clearer to me that I would often go to bed with someone for the cuddling that came afterward. I think there are probably a lot of gay men who secretly embrace the idea of a more subdued sexual life-style. On the other hand, I'm the first to put up my dukes when I hear someone use AIDS to disparage the very real pleasures of promiscuity. It's enormously important that we don't let this epidemic turn us into Calvinists. I think we're liberating the world with our ideas about sex. We're putting sex in its place; we're not making it so goddamned important. We're not murdering each other over it like those straight suburban couples you read about.

Has this changed your values about life and death?

No. I've always felt that I could go tomorrow. And that feeling shapes my approach to everything. I'm usually pretty comfortable around people who are dying—they don't play games, and they have a marvelous way with irony. I look for those qualities in everyone I meet, and I almost never find them.

What do you mean, "a way with irony"?

Well . . . a friend of mine, for instance, a guy with pneumocystis pneumonia, asked me to go with him to his lover's mother's funeral. The mother, who was a California aristocrat, had never permitted my friend in the house. Now she was dead, and her son's lover had a sentence—as he put it—of six months, but he wanted to go to her funeral to provide support for his lover. Now, that's about as fraught with irony as you can get. We winked and grinned at each other throughout the service, and I couldn't help thinking what all those tight-assed Episcopalians would think if they knew that a man with AIDS was in their midst, looking so eminently respectable.

The priest who officiated over the funeral came up afterward and spoke to the two lovers and said, "Oh, you must come over for dinner one night," and after the priest left I said, "What was that all about?" and my friend replied, "Well, Father John and his lover just invited us to dinner." I wasn't sure I had heard him correctly. "His *lover?*" And my friend grinned and said, "Yes, Father Frank over there!"

Well, we just roared. I mean, here were these two priests in their clerical collars, they both had upper-class heterosexual parishioners, and they had been living together for years, and one of them had just presided over the funeral of a woman who wouldn't let her son's male lover into the house. Hypocrisy in full, glorious bloom. You see a lot of that when you're gay . . . and even more, I think, when you're facing death.

Has this changed your attitudes about society and gay freedom?

Well, it just means we're going to have to fight even harder to achieve visibility. Hollywood, for instance, had a period when AIDS caused them to back away like crazy from gay subject matter. That's when Steven Carrington turned straight on "Dynasty." Now he's going gay again, so I guess the worst is over.

How effective do you think the biological family has been in dealing with this epidemic?

It really depends on the family in question. The parents of one of my friends gave him nothing but love and support up until his death. They were sort of liberal to begin with, though. Another friend, who has KS, wasn't allowed to go home to his father's funeral in Kansas. So the reaction ranges from heart-warming to heartbreaking, depending upon the wisdom of the particular family.

What about the effectiveness of organized medicine?

I'm really not in a position to judge. I believe enough in human greed, though, to think that they must be trying to find a cure. It's going to mean the Nobel Prize for someone.

How about psychologists? Any impressions about how psychologists have dealt with this?

No. And I really don't care. I stopped listening to psychologists years ago. If I had listened to them when I was a teenager I would have had electrodes attached to my balls. I have never felt that psychologists were the answer to anything.

What about gay psychologists?

Not too long ago, I said to a friend (unfortunately in front of someone who turned out to be a gay psychologist) that the only thing more fucked up than a gay priest is a gay psychologist. I don't want to be held responsible for that remark, but it may give you an idea as to my general response to those institutions. To me, to be gay is to live a life without rules, and psychologists have rules, priests have rules, lawyers have rules, and they have to play within that framework, and I don't. I don't want to have to play within that framework. I make that position fairly clear in a little presentation I do from time to time called "Mondo Homo," in which I read from psychologists on the subject of homosexuality throughout the twentieth century. You hear the most absurd imaginable things.

Like what?

Well, as late as the '50s there were psychologists who were saying that men like to suck on each other's dicks because it reminds them of sucking milk from our mother's breast. Well, please, why do we like to chew on men's tits, then? Because it reminds us of our mother's pussy? I have no idea what they're talking about, and they don't either. There was another body of thought which maintained that a man's ass in tight pants reminded us of the jiggling of a woman's breasts. I mean, tits were very, very big with these guys. *Nobody* was supposed to admire a man's ass in those days, not even the women. Psychiatry, in my view, is just society's clumsy way of deciding what's normal, and that means somebody's gonna get burned.

What is your impression about organized religion and their response to this?

At the risk of proclaiming the obvious, I think the fundamentalists are anything but Christlike on the subject of AIDS. They've simply used it as an example of the uncleanliness of homosexuals, which would be regarded as nothing short of monstrous if they had done the same thing with blacks and sickle-cell anemia. If Jerry Falwell had said, "See, those niggers are dirty, just like we told you all along," there would have been a deafening outcry from the liberals in the country. Yet, that's what they've tried to do to us, and where are our defenders?

Not long ago, I did a radio talk show here on which a woman caller from Sacramento told me that homosexuals deserve to die as long as they continue to "do those unnatural things." I explained to her as calmly as possible—which was not very calmly, I'm afraid—that sex is the way in which AIDS is spread, *not* the cause of it. The distinction eluded her completely. This was God saying, "Knock it off, boys," and that's all there was to it.

What about the federal government? What's your analysis of how they've responded?

Well, there *has* been more money pledged for it recently—just about the time they realized that heterosexuals were also susceptible to the disease. There again, using the sickle-cell anemia analogy, what if they had said, "Sickle-cell anemia is a threat to the general welfare, because white people might eventually get it." Imagine the horror with which such a remark would be met!

How about the mainstream press? Any impressions about the way they've dealt with it?

Sure—they ignored it until they realized the magnitude of it and were so embarrassed over having ignored it that they bombarded the public with it and scared them to death. That gave them a brand new thing to write about: "AIDS Hysteria." Most people are enormously naive about the ways in which the press manipulates them. I've been a reporter—I know. I know how the whole procedure works. You write a story, and you get a reaction to it, then you get two factions warring, and you go say, "He said this about you, so what do you have to say about that?"

Do you think the bathhouses should be closed?

No.

Why not?

Because it's not *where* you do it, it's what you do, and any gay man who lives in this town knows that there's just as many exotic sex practices going on in any house on that hillside as in a cubicle at Eighth and Howard. And there's also a question of freedom involved here. It breaks my heart that there are men who go out in the midst of this epidemic and have sex as if there were no tomorrow, because I do think that's a destructive form of behavior, but they're going to do that whether there's a bathhouse or not.

Why do you think they're doing that?

I wish I knew. I think there's a—at the risk of sounding like a psychologist—I think a lot of people have their whole identity tied up in their sexual behavior and that their sense of acceptance comes from that. They've never learned to be peaceful with themselves.

What can be done, then, to educate these people?

I don't know—short of dragging them into the AIDS wards and having them see for themselves. I'm utterly mystified by the apparent indifference of some people.

You mentioned earlier that your own sexual identity has evolved in such a way that it's not so attached to sexual behavior. Can you elaborate on that?

Well, it's just that I've learned to get genuine satisfaction from the kind of blanketing gay love that I give to my friends and that I get back from them, a sense of brotherhood and community that runs hand in hand with a healthy appreciation of sex. It's funny—you hear gay men reminiscing about the old days at the bathhouses. But it really *was* different in the early '70s. There was a kind of community. I think maybe some of the old hippie thing was still around. At any rate, as the bathhouse and bars became more institutionalized, they became lonelier places, and much less fulfilling. So maybe there are people who keep going back, expecting to get some sort of fulfillment, and they never really get it.

So maybe they're still going not so much out of self-hatred and a fatalistic outlook as to seek that sort of camaraderie.

Yes. That's exactly why I used to go. It was a club for me, a peaceful, secret place where you could put the world aside for a while. It could be quite extraordinary. I'd come out of it at three o'clock in the morning and walk home feeling like a million bucks. I had spiritual feelings at the baths. This is tough to talk about, because people who haven't experienced it—especially straight people—think you're out of your mind. But that's the way it was for me. I felt closer to God at the baths. I don't feel that so much anymore, so I don't go anymore, at least not with any kind of frequency.

How do you think the AIDS epidemic will affect society's treatment of homosexuals?

A backlash, you mean?

Yes.

You know, I'm asked about backlashes a lot, and I've gotten rather numb to the question. We haven't had the frontlash yet, have we? As homosexuals, we *begin* with the understanding that society is going to fight us every inch of the way. We can't waste our energy anticipating future resistance. It's tough enough keeping our own goals in view.

Do you think that there's any opportunity here to broaden our concept of humanity, so that we don't see homosexuals and heterosexuals as being distinct, but sexuality as being inclusive?

That's always been my dream. And it drives me crazy that

almost everything conspires against that, including most gay people. We are all too willing to be ghettoized. Look at my own line of work. The way the publishing industry has dealt with the rise in books with gay subject matter is to create an entirely separate genre, a separate shelf in the bookstores. There's no way I'm writing just for gay people. I want my message to reach the world at large. But this literary segregation has happened to every writer who dares to question the white, straight, male-dominated society we live in. The women have their own shelf, the blacks have their own shelf, the gays have their own shelf—as if we are in no way connected to Norman Mailer and Saul Bellow and the so-called mainstream literature of this country. What keeps us from sticking those guys on a Jewish Interest shelf?

Is there a way for us to expose somehow the howl of oppression that keeps these different groups from coming together?

Well, in the first place, I've always been annoyed by the term "minority." What the hell does that mean? This country is nothing but minorities. America is supposed to be a celebration of the fact that a human being is a human being. The very term "minority" suggests some sort of lesser consideration, and I think the civil rights movement did us all a disservice by inventing the concept in the first place. I cringe when I hear gay leaders say we deserve minority consideration like anybody else. I mean, fuck that, I'm a human being like anybody else; I'm an American like anybody else. I have a right to lead my life the way I want to lead it.

If you were just now coming out, how do you think the AIDS epidemic would affect you?

I'm sure it would be much harder. I'll always be glad I had

seven or eight years to explore my sexuality absolutely free from fear.

What did you learn in those seven or eight years?

Oh, that sex was a source of enormous pleasure and comfort, that it was no big deal, that it was no substitute for true affection and love, but could go hand in hand with it or be completely separate from it and still be fun.

13

The Horrible
and the Wonderful

Linda Maxey

Linda Maxey is a counseling coordinator for services provided to AIDS patients on Ward 5B at San Francisco General Hospital by the Shanti Project. Her background is in nursing. She is a thirty-six-year-old heterosexual woman who lives in San Francisco and is in excellent health. Linda has worked with death and dying issues within a hospital setting for several years.

I

When did you first learn about AIDS?

I've been with the Shanti Project for about two years. I joined in February 1982. At that time there wasn't that much about AIDS, but Jim Geary and another counselor were leading a support group for people with AIDS. A psychologist from U.C. had contacted Shanti and wanted Shanti to become their resource and referral center for people with AIDS. He was aware that there was a growing number of people. He was working at the KS clinic at U.C. and was aware that there was a growing need for support for people with AIDS. That's how Shanti got involved. His name was Paul Dague, and he came and contacted us to do support groups and that's sort of how we began, and then, as the epidemic kept increasing, we started becoming more and more involved to the point where what's happened recently is that we've had to limit our services just to people with AIDS, primarily because we're city funded to meet the needs. The city also then came to us when they were trying to coordinate services in the city and wanted us to be the organization to meet psychosocial needs of people with AIDS. I was on the board of directors at the time and also involved here and became involved pretty actively in what was happening with AIDS.

So your information about AIDS came directly from being involved with people who had the illness?

Right, right. I went to several seminars and a lot of workshops that have been put on to get more medical information, and I also did public speaking. As a volunteer, I had clients who had AIDS. I was one of the facilitators for the volunteer counselor training in July. This will be the first time I will not be in a training, but I'm probably going to show up. I'm hooked. I'm a junkie. (They laugh.) I really love doing the trainings, but doing the work here, I've had to quit a little bit of it. Cliff Morrison, the clinical coordinator here, who had also been in the Shanti Project—I trained him—was setting up this unit in the hospital. He came to Shanti and wanted to contract with us to staff the unit with counselors seven days a week, and wanted me to coordinate that. So that's how I got here.

Without using the term *AIDS*, would you describe how you see this illness?

I would describe it as a deficiency in the immune system

that leaves people open and vulnerable to secondary opportunistic infections and to different types of cancers and lymphomas that seem to be somehow related to immune depression. I think there's some agent or agents that cause this, and that's where it gets real nebulous as to what really results in people having AIDS. In working in this area, I think the initial stereotypes of the people who get this disease have proven not to hold a lot of water. And the more I see, the more I realize we don't know. I think everybody's looking for what we know to try to find that safe place to hang onto, and when you work with it day to day, you realize that there are so many things that don't fall into what people think they know about this.

For example?

For example, people who have had very rare sexual experiences. We're seeing one man lately who claims never to have taken in semen in the last five years, and is not an IV drug user. Where does he get it? People that are real monogamous, you know. I think he's still in a relationship, but he just doesn't fall into that category, is real health oriented and all that. I sense sometimes it's like a cold. Do you have to be exposed three times before you get it, or is once enough? I mean, there are all those kinds of questions. I don't know.

How do you perceive your own risk for contracting AIDS?

Logically, I think I'm at low risk in some ways. I've had sexual experiences with a bisexual or predominantly—I don't know what he calls it. I've always wondered. (They laugh.)

He's a human.

He's a human, I know! That whole thing, the categories, I don't know. But he's in a high-risk category, and we had a sexual relationship two years ago for a while, and where that puts me, I don't know. I don't think about it a lot. I don't feel at risk working with the people here on the unit. My life-style right now puts me at very low risk. I've never done IV drugs and I also, right now, am not having a lot of sexual relationships, so I feel like I'm not at such a high risk.

And yet there are times where the irrational part of it comes up. I mean, I sit here and I hug these men and kiss them. There's one man I get real close to; I spend a tremendous amount of time with him. I never was concerned about risk or feeling any of it, and all of a sudden one day he laid his sweaty little head on my shoulder and I leaned over and kissed him and I could feel the perspiration. It hit me then, like "Oh, my!" It was totally irrational, you know. It didn't have a thing to do with what I know about transmissibility. But it was just that instant where it hits you and it doesn't always make sense when it does.

How much confidence do you have in the CDC's description of transmissibility and risk?

I know that it's not casually transmitted. That part I do know. How exactly it's transmitted becomes a little more confusing. I believe that there's been epidemiological evidence, which is where all of our information about transmissibility really comes from right now. I do believe it requires really intimate contact through either needle sharing or exchange of body fluids or blood products. What body fluids is another question. I trust that they are getting as much evidence and making as valuable assumptions about it as possible, given that we can't isolate the agent at this point.

**How do you perceive the risk for people who have AIDS
of contracting other infections?**

I think the risk is great.

How is it that they might contract those?

Well, pneumocystis is in our environment. At least forty to
fifty percent of us currently have the pneumocystis organism
in our bodies. The problem is that a lot of these infections that
people get are infections that are currently already in their system, and it's only when the immune system gets so low that
their body's normal mechanisms can't fight it off that infections
will take over. So, for a large portion, I believe that they've
already got the illness. It's a matter of "Can their immune system stay at a level where they can continue to fight it off?" I
don't know how it is or why it is that some people end up with
pneumocystis and others don't, and why some end up with
cryptococcal meningitis and others don't. How you get a specific infection, I really don't know.

**How much neurological impairment do you see in people
with AIDS?**

We're starting to see more. We're currently starting to see
people getting toxoplasmosis, cryptococcal meningitis, and
lymphomas. We're starting to see more "neuro" problems. I
think we're just starting to see more, period, so all of it's going
to increase.

**Is it conceivable to you that it's a neurological illness that
then would send out improper signals to the rest of the body,
particularly the immune system? That it could have its gene-
sis, in fact, in the neurological system?**

That sounds feasible to me. It would have to be something that starts without people developing neurological problems, because that isn't the most common presenting problem. So it is feasible that if it's a virus, it affects whatever portion regulates the immune system. But the immune system is so unknown. There are 40 million links in the immune system. Which link is it, or is it several, or what is it that results in deficiency?

Are you familiar with any of the similarities to Agent Orange?

No, I don't really know much about Agent Orange.

How do you control for your own risk in contracting the illness while you're working with people?

In my interactions with clients, I don't think I do too much. I don't really have that much contact. I'm not working as a nurse on the unit here; therefore, I don't start IVs and I'm not at such risk of getting stuck with contaminated needles. I don't think that I really take a lot of precautions. I wash my hands. I think that's the thing that most of us do on the unit that feels like the most appropriate thing to do. If I empty someone's urinal of if I help someone off a bedpan, I wash my hands. I've cleaned up people who've been incontinent, and when I do that I wear gloves. If I'm cleaning body secretions up, I wear gloves, and I wash my hands before and after seeing patients if I'm having physical contact with them. If someone has an active cough, we sometimes wear masks, but that's not common.

How would you recommend people with AIDS controlling their own risk for contracting other illnesses while in one another's company?

I think if someone has active pneumocystis—we've had support groups where people have been in different places. If someone is newly diagnosed with pneumocystis and has an active cough, I think that the best thing to do is for either them to wear a mask or for the other people to wear a mask, while they're actively coughing. Once they're not coughing, I don't think there's any risk. People get to be friends here and come and visit all the time. If someone with AIDS is visiting a friend of theirs who's just diagnosed with pneumocystis and is actively coughing, we'll suggest that they wear a mask to protect themselves. Otherwise, there's probably not that much in terms of just casual contact. In terms of intimate contact, I think it's true for every person, I don't think it matters whether you have AIDS or you don't. I think everybody needs to take the same precautions. I don't think that there's any difference.

And those precautions—you're referring to the safe sex precautions?

Right. Not exchanging body fluids, not sharing needles, that kind of thing.

Is the risk of contracting AIDS any different from other kinds of risks that you take in your life? For example, the risk of being in a car accident or having a heart attack or taking a gamble in Reno?

Well, I think that there's some degree of more control over it in some ways, in a car accident. I mean, in a car accident, you can kind of control in that you shouldn't drive when you're drinking and you need to know good driving techniques, but there's always that craziness that can happen that's totally out of your control. I think those elements are also in AIDS, to some degree, but I think there are things that we can do to make changes in our lives to decrease the risk of AIDS.

What is is that you're gaining by interacting with AIDS patients?

For me personally? Oh, I get a *lot* out of this work. A *lot*. I get a lot from the people with AIDS. They're incredible people. There's such an openness a lot of times. It's like going through a crisis with somebody; you become closer as a result of it than you do if you're just chatting in a bar and in common interactions. I think there's an intimacy there just by nature of the crisis, by nature of what's happening, a bond.

The community's incredible, and here on 5B we've just become close—to each other, to the patients. The boundaries of nurse/patient, counselor/patient get real nebulous. People become friends. I have people that I've gotten to know simply because they have AIDS, but they've become my friend and there are many times I don't relate to them as a person with AIDS. They're just my pinochle partner! (Laughs.) My cruise-mate, whatever.

I go to the beach and AIDS doesn't exist. It'll come up, though, all of a sudden, when we're going to go for a walk on the beach and the person I'm with puts their pants on because they're self-conscious about the lesions on their legs. Then it comes back to me that, yes, he does have AIDS, but for the most part, he's just my buddy.

What are the kinds of emotional experiences you have had through dealing with AIDS?

(Sighs.) I've felt everything: angry, hurt, sad, fear—I've felt every conceivable emotion. I get angry at homophobic responses to this, I get tired of having to defend it. I used to do a lot of public speaking before I got this job, and trying to help other people understand what it's like to have AIDS, what it's like to be gay and have this disease, what all this is about—

and you work so hard doing that that it seems endless. So I get angry at that: When are people just going to wake up and see that this is not a gay disease, it's a human issue? You know, I get real frustrated with that, so I get angry. I get angry at people who want simplistic answers to this, who want to close the bathhouses and feel that's the way to stay safe.

I get angry and I also get sad. I see the agony behind that also. Those people are in agony. They're not jerks. They're just people who don't know how to live with this kind of fear constantly, who don't know how to be anymore, who don't know how to be intimate and be a sexual being. I see the grief; I get sad when I see the grief in the community over a loss of being able to be sexually free, and also the grief over the fact that this is touching everybody's lives.

It's not here on 5B anymore. When we first opened this unit, it seemed to be the patients on the unit, but we all have friends who have AIDS, and we've watched our friends die as well as the patients here. It feels like being in a war at times. We're looking at the staff support. My fear is, these are incredible people doing this work; how long can they do it? Then you get all the politics, and in that—forget that! I mean, that just is absurd to me. I mean, people are dying and then other people are out there arguing over money and craziness.

The infighting within the gay community with the newspapers disturbs me greatly, too.

Right. I get furious. I get furious over that. That just angers me to no end. Shanti is not perfect, neither is the AIDS Foundation, neither is the AIDS Fund, neither is any one of us as individuals. But God, you know, you can't keep trying to do the work and also have to respond to media attacks and everybody's self-interests. That kind of stuff drives me crazy.

I wish all those people that were so eager to attack people

in the paper would just come over here and work for a couple of days. Let's get to the heart of what we're really talking about. All those people that sit up there and bitch about money and the federal government, let's watch someone die here together and then you tell me about money! That kind of stuff really gets frustrating.

How would you characterize your own emotional maturity in the last year?

I think I've grown a lot. It's pushed my boundaries, it's pushed my thinking I know anything to the limit, thinking I understand life and death and why an epidemic when so many young people are dying. To be with people that are facing this crisis you have to let go of your ego a lot, you have to totally let go of what you think you know. I think I've learned to live with uncertainty and learned to hang out in that space. Learning to be a good follower in a dance where the music changes rapidly. You know, I feel like I'm working with people, they're leading, I'm following, I'm just trying to keep up and hang in there, and sometimes it's a waltz and sometimes it's a polka.

Has your life changed any since this?

Oh, my God. Don't ask me that question! (Laughs.) Oh, my God. What life? That's probably the heart of it. We were talking about this in our support group the other day. This work isn't a nine-to-five, Monday-through-Friday office job where you can leave your work there and go home. It hits the core of all of us; it makes us look at all the issues that everybody puts off till they're seventy or eighty years old, and we're being asked to look at that now. I've grown spiritually, I've grown emotionally, and I have also—I don't know how to explain it—

Are there any particular evaluations that you've done of things that you do?

My values are different. My house is a complete shambles. (Laughs.) I mean, it is a *mess!* And my priorities have changed. I need more time to myself now. I can't keep up the same social life I did before. I don't make all the parties and do all that kind of thing, because I need some quiet time and my own space more. I'm learning—for the first time, I've been forced to learn how to deal with getting replenished and renurtured in a way that I've never had to do before. So I'm looking at that, like meditation and yoga and exercise. It's emotionally challenging and rewarding.

How has it changed your values about life and death?

I used to sit and think I knew what I was going to be doing in five years. When I joined Shanti, I was going to do it until I got into graduate school in September. I took my GREs in January and I was just going to fill in time, right? (Laughs.) That was three years ago! And then when I thought, "Well, maybe my time in Shanti is almost up," then this happened and I was into doing this job. I've given up looking at or worrying about the future. I think I'm more in the moment than I've ever been. I've had to let go of thinking that my social obligations—I've let go of guilt about not keeping them. And just not worrying so much about all those kinds of crazy things. I don't worry about my house being dirty as much.

II

Has being involved with AIDS changed your values about gay liberation?

When I first got involved in Shanti, I had worked with gay men—I was a nurse doing nursing before this, and I had worked with gay men as patients, but I really didn't know them much, other than parties we'd go to, but as far as a personal friendship, I really didn't have any close gay friends. And through doing this and through being in this group, I've developed a lot of friendships with gay men. I didn't know much about the different types of life-styles and about the gay community when I started doing this, and I've learned a lot.

I feel like I've also developed a lot of nonjudgmentalness. You know, I don't have a strong judgment about any particular life-style being right or wrong. Now I have concerns about people being at risk and I want them to be safe, but I don't have a judgment about any particular sexual practice being ridiculous. I don't have judgments about bathhouses. Is this going to go in the book?

Sure it is.

Uh-oh! (Laughs.) Well, one time I got curious about bathhouses. I was actually getting jealous about bathhouses. Having been in the straight scene for a while, the bar scene wasn't that much fun. I was talking to a friend of mine one night and I said, "You know, I think you gay men have it made. You've got these bathhouses where you can go and you can have sex, you can be intimate, you can get hugged, you can get touched, and you don't have to play all the games. You don't have to wake up in the morning with this person and say, 'Oh, my God, now what do I do?'"

And so I went to this bathhouse with this friend of mine and it was a real interesting and wonderful experience. I found that the code of ethics there was higher than in bars, in many ways. People didn't assume they owned you because they bought you this drink, and if you said no, there wasn't that "hurtness," that rejection, all that—there was just such an ease about it.

There were a lot of things that I could see being very wonderful and enticing about it, and I can also see the dilemmas with it and problems with it. I think you can get hooked into that so that you don't form intimate relationships because it's so easy to have contact and it's real safe and then it's over and you don't have to work through problems in relationships, or difficulties, or iron out those hard times.

So I see good points and bad points to everybody's life-style. And I thought, "Jeez, you know, if bathhouses were as readily accepted in the straight community, I'd probably be in them all the time!" (Laughs.) I just thought it would be so much easier at the end of the day to go to a bathhouse than a bar, you know. I just thought it sounded pretty appealing to me. And it was interesting because after that I did think about that one night.

Some of them are very beautiful. I mean, I think that people think that they're trashy and sleazy and greasy, and I think there probably are some like that, but some of them are incredibly wonderful.

After that, though, I thought about it. I wish I had the courage to go into the bathhouses by myself, and then also AIDS came up and I realized that even if there were more freedom right now, I don't know if I would feel safe going. I think that what's happening now is that we've gotten this fear out there, "AIDS is here, watch out, there's risk," all these fear-oriented words, but what's not happening is helping people learn enjoyable ways of having sex with all those limitations that need to happen right now. We've said, "Here are the limitations," but that's much easier said than doing it.

It's the same issue for women and birth control, I think. Over the years, it's always been something that's been very difficult for women in that condoms are not always the most pleasurable thing in the world; just having to do it takes away spontaneity, whether it's condoms, the diaphragm, foam, or whatever. The pill and the IUD were wonderful options, but for many women those aren't options.

They're dangerous.

Right, and for me personally they're not options. So then it became, "How do you have sex, make it enjoyable, and not worry about getting pregnant?" And you need a partner that is going to help you with that; you can't just do it yourself. So I think that's what men right now are trying to figure out: how to be safe and how to have it be enjoyable, and what if your partner doesn't think that's enjoyable, or what if—you know, who does the burden fall on? It should fall on everybody, but it doesn't always.

This is an interesting parallel that you've drawn between the experience of birth control and the experience of safe sex. I think there are other parallels that might be drawn in other things that gay men can now learn from women in terms of health care. After reading the book, *For Her Own Good*, it became very clear to me that we had a lot to learn from women. Are gay men really learning anything from women and from the women's movement about how to take charge of their own health care?

I don't know what they're learning from the women's movement, to be honest. I guess, having been a part of it, I'm not even sure if I have a scope of what I know about health care, being a woman. I've been a nurse, so it's hard for me to separate what I know about health care from being a nurse or a woman or whatever.

You're an R.N.?

Uh-huh. I think the women's movement became a real standing up and saying, "We're going to take charge of this and we're *not* going to be subjected to other people's opinions or statements about women's bodies." I know I always used to have incredibly awful premenstrual problems and would go to a male gynecologist who'd tell me it was all in my head.

Finally I got so angry at one of them, I said, "When you have your first period, then you come to me and you tell me what it's like," and until then, I didn't trust him. And I always felt degraded and put down, and I think women decided we're going to take care of ourselves, and we're not going to buy all that, and we know better.

I think that people with AIDS—it's the first time in my whole nursing career that I think I've seen such a cohesive group of people stand up and demand their rights. I don't know if they learned that from the women's movement or not; I'm not sure. But I think that being a predominantly male population, they're more outspoken and they've taken a lot more initiative to get what they need. They've demanded people that care and see what's going on. They've worked incredibly hard to reach out to the community, to educate people, to dispel the gap or to bridge the gap, and so I think they're a very cohesive, outspoken group who's going to make some decisions on their own about health care, who've made changes in health care.

I think that people with AIDS have made dramatic changes. I've seen it here on 5B. Questioning doctors, questioning authority, and also working with them to help *them*. I've seen patients help their doctors in dealing with this. It's pretty amazing to watch.

Do you notice some patients doing better than others, and do you notice a pattern in any of their dealing with the illness that might determine how their prognosis is?

(Pause.) I think if you're looking at the goal of getting better, the goal of getting rid of the illness, I'm not sure. If the goal is in the process of having the illness, in going through the process, I think there are some things that make a difference.

I think support makes a tremendous difference. I think dealing with anything in an isolated situation, alone, feeling like you can't reach out to anyone and no one's there for you, makes the process of it much worse. Possibly it makes the outcome worse, but I don't think I can make a definitive statement about that.

I've seen people who've come from the place of deciding at the beginning that they're going to be very positive about this. They're going to work on increasing self-affirmations, increasing visualizations, to do healings, to try combining alternatives with traditional. I've seen people make all kinds of choices about what they're going to do. I've seen people give up smoking and drinking and changing life-styles dramatically.

And I think support's made a big difference in having that ability to do that. And I've seen people do that and die, quicker than other people that continue with alcohol and drugs and not taking the best possible care of themselves.

In the outcome of the illness, life or death, I don't know that it makes a difference. But in the journey, I think there are a lot of things that make a difference. The journey with someone else is easier than alone. Being able to be open to asking for help is hard for a lot of men, and I've seen people break through that a lot, sometimes not until right at the end.

I think meeting other people that are in the same situation, support groups, and knowing that there's someone else there in the same situation is helpful. I think being in a supportive environment—you know, that can be interpersonal relationships at home, living situations, formal organizational support, whatever—and not having to deal with "judgmentalness" of other people helps a lot. Self-esteem—I think self-esteem makes a big difference.

What about in contracting the illness? Do you think that there's a pre-AIDS personality?

Oh, gosh, I get really angry when I hear that! (Laughs.) I have a hard time with that, and that's my own personal opinion about it. I remember when people were trying to come up with the "type A" personality for people that had heart attacks, and I was working in a coronary care unit. I thought that did a disservice to people in high-stress jobs who may never come down with a heart attack and also did a disservice to people who came down with them and couldn't figure out why and thought maybe they had a "hidden type A."

(Laughs.)

You know, and then they'd start questioning themselves so much, and I thought, "Don't. Forget that." So I feel like there's a lot to be said about the mind-body connection and I think it's so far removed from what we know now that to make statements about it can really be a disservice to people—that idea that you created your own illness. The idea that if you create it, you should be able to get rid of it. I've seen people struggle with that to the point where it is a disservice to them or it hinders them. It lays guilt on people. It comes out real simplistically, but it's incredibly complex.

If there is indeed any truth to that at all, it's not something that people have a handle on now, to be able to use. So I caution people against that. I've seen people try positive thinking and then when it fails, they feel not only are they faced with their illness getting worse, but they feel like a failure in addition.

Exactly.

And that breaks my heart to watch that. So I have strong reactions to that.

III

I'd like to ask you about the effectiveness of certain systems and institutions, and we'll start with the biological family. You probably see a lot of interaction between family members and people with AIDS. How would you characterize that?

Well, there's a range, from wonderful to terrible. I've seen some people whose families won't have anything to do with them and they die alone, without having much contact with their family. Then I've seen families who have dealt with all kinds of incredibly heavy and difficult issues in a real short amount of time and have risen beyond all expectations. I don't know if *I* could have dealt with it so well. Who had to find out for the first time that not only is their son gay, but that he also has a life-threatening illness and he's in the hospital and he's not doing well.

Is that a large determinant in how they're going to react, how they've dealt with or known about or not known about their son's sexuality before?

I don't think so. I think that—well, boy, I don't know. That issue has a lot of different levels of implications. There are times when I've seen families who feel like, "If only I had done something for him not to be gay, then he wouldn't have gotten this. And they deal with that, feeling guilty. Parents' natural instinct is to protect their children, and they feel like they should have taken care of them better, and at that point they end up feeling guilty because they think they should have done something so he wouldn't be gay, because that's why he got this disease. And we have to work through that understanding.

And I think what happens here, this magic, is that parents will come here, have to deal with those issues about finding out their son's gay at the same time as they have to deal with the issues about the possibility of losing him, and what they see here is the acceptance. And that helps them through that feeling like their son's gay, so he's—whatever their judgments about gay people are.

They see us caring for them, they see the interactions here, people treated as people, and the issue about him being gay somehow just gets taken care of. I think they see that we value their son and love him as a person, and how wonderful he is, and that his sexuality doesn't matter, that he's a human being that's incredibly wonderful. So some of that, I think just by being in this situation where they witness other people loving their son and caring for him and not worried about his sexuality helps. They see other parents with their sons. So I think some of that gets taken care of just by role modeling or whatever you want to call it.

Sometimes we have to work very hard on their misconceptions about being gay. I have one mother—this sounds crazy when I say it, but listening to her, I can understand. Her son had had some psychiatric problems in the past, and she thought that being gay caused brain damage. She just knew he had trouble with relating at times. Maybe it was that being gay caused brain damage. And it wasn't brain damage and it wasn't being gay. She just didn't have any idea what all that was about.

We had to do a lot of education around that to her: the difference between brain damage and an emotional problem; someone having a history of needing psychiatric support having nothing to do with being gay; that people that are gay have the same problem and people that are gay don't, so it doesn't have anything to do with that. Helping her understand that she doesn't have control over her son's preferences around sexuality took away some of her sense of feeling responsible.

So sometimes it just requires education. I think that often-times parents will also feel guilty if they weren't able to handle their son coming out to them about being gay. Now he's dying, and maybe they have not been able to be there as much during his life as they would have wished, and now there's no more second chance. It can be devastating. And I've seen them work through a lot of that in an incredibly short amount of time.

I've seen families have to be closeted. That's been some-thing I wasn't aware of before. A mother and father who have known about their son being gay since he was twenty, who loved him dearly. He was an amazing twenty-four-year-old. At twenty he came out being gay, left the navy, brought his lover home, and moved in with his parents. I asked him what that was like, and he said, "Well, you know, they sat there and after a couple of weeks they said, 'Well, there's not really much difference between you and us.'"

(Laughs.)

And then the issue was no problem at all. But when he got AIDS, the mother couldn't tell her friends what he had because her friends had so many judgments. To protect her son, be-cause she wasn't going to let anybody say anything bad about him, she had to become closeted regarding what was happen-ing with her son. And I think that happens to families that I think we sometimes aren't as aware of.

True.

And people were telling her, "Be careful; don't kiss him," and she said, "If my son's going to die, he's not going to die without me hugging and kissing him."

How about lovers?

Lovers vary, too. Some of them can't handle it and they pull away. Not because they're bad people, but they just can't handle the possibility of someone they love so much, watching them deteriorate and die. And we try and support them in that respect, too. I think lovers oftentimes feel—as do families, as do roommates, as do friends—they have to be the strong ones, they've got to be there for the other person.

We try and let them know that they, too, deserve and need support. This isn't a process that just the person with AIDS is going through, it's their process, too, and they are every bit as deserving and needing of support. We try and encourage them to get that. We're here for them as much as we are for the one who's got AIDS.

Lovers—there are all kinds of dynamics that come up. When families come from across the country and arrive on the scene, the lover's been the one—or the roommate, oftentimes—the one who's been driving them to the clinic three times a week, the one who's been doing the cooking, getting the groceries, helping take care of them at home, fixing their meals, then the mother arrives. Well, mothers, being mothers, want to take over, and so sometimes we have to work out, you know, we've got two mothers now. (Laughs.)

Helping mothers and families see that their son has another family here and that they can work together, that oftentimes is a real relief to them. The lover is oftentimes the one that puts the family up, takes them around the city, helps bring them to the hospital, picks them up at the airport, takes them back to the airport. And they usually can work that out.

It just means sometimes we end up being facilitators in a crazy situation initially and trying to validate the place each person's at and also helping them see where everybody's at, so that there's not a conflict but a cooperative way of everybody getting their needs met.

How do you think organized medicine has reacted to this?

Are we organized? (They laugh.) Organized medicine . . . (Pause.) Again, I think the people with AIDS have forced changes. They're about to say, "All your stuff doesn't fit anymore," you know, and they've said, "You've got to make changes; this isn't going to work," and I think that they have done a lot to get those changes made.

There still needs to be more. I'm not sure what it all is. I mean, organized medicine—we have a big gap right now in that when people leave the hospital—we're talking about a lot of people who are single and who live alone. We're not talking about the 1900s where there were three generations standing around someone when they were ill to take care and pick up the other part of the burdens of life, financially and roles and getting the chores done.

So what's missing now is that people will come into the hospital and they're not just a person that's staying in a house. They're a person that has to figure out how they're going to get groceries and how they're going to get food and how they're going to deal with life at home, you know, and I think we're starting to recognize that you can't just see somebody in a clinic and send them home without worrying about what they're going home to.

I feel like a lot of efforts are starting to be made to have more consciousness about discharge planning, about "What's your life like at home?", helping to figure out ways to make that better so they don't have to come into the hospital as often. I think that's still a gap, but it's being worked on and I think people with AIDS are making them say, "Hey, do you want to know why I'm losing weight? I haven't had anybody to help get me groceries or fix my meals."

So I think there's an awareness about a whole person, the wholeness of people, that's occurred here, particularly. At the hospital there never used to be—there was no precedent for this. There wasn't even an oncology unit where the issues of life and death and the realities of people being sick and chronically sick over a long period of time had to be looked at, and I think that there have been major changes made here along those lines.

What about public health?

The Public Health Department in San Francisco, to me, is pretty impressive. I've been amazed at the coordination of services. I go to the AIDS Coordinating Committee meeting once a month. That was designed to see that all needs were being met, that duplication of services wasn't occurring, and look at where the gaps are and figure out ways to fill those gaps.

And I think that's what's really essential in health care, period, whether it's at the public health level, whether it's even on a unit level: coordination of services. It's a team effort; it's not the doctors doing their thing and the nurses doing their thing and us doing ours with no communication. It's got to be a cooperative effort.

How does homeopathic medicine fit into all that?

I think with AIDS, more and more doctors are recognizing

they don't have the answers; they certainly don't know what's going on all the time. I think that when people ask, "What about vitamins?", a lot more doctors are saying, "Well, I don't want you to think that that's the cure for this, but it isn't going to hurt you. As long as it's monitored, try it. Try visualization, try all these other things."

I think there's been more of a willingness to expand preconceived notions that the traditional medical model is the only way. It certainly hasn't solved this yet. And here we are pretty open to that. There's an alternative therapy clinic where people can get visualization, assistance in doing that, or self-hypnosis, acupressure—so there is more of an incorporation.

But these two systems seem somehow still to be separate. The homeopathic community doesn't sit down with the traditional medical community. I haven't seen a lot of that.

What kind of response have you seen from psychologists to the AIDS epidemic?

We have a psychiatrist here who's used as a liaison consulting person. He was Cliff's preference from the Psychiatry Department and he is wonderful. He's a wonderful man and we've worked well together.

Shanti being here is a precedent. Never before has a volunteer organization been asked to staff the unit of a hospital in a traditional health-care setting. There was some reluctance, I think, on the part of Psychiatry. Psychiatry's always been the ones that took care of anything that falls under the category of an emotion. If it's not in your body, you know, totally body-related, they would always ship it off to Psychiatry.

Well, facing life-threatening illness isn't a psychiatric problem, it's a human problem, so there was some question about how we would integrate services. It's worked out very well. All the people doing psychosocial support meet once a week, and that includes the psychiatrists, myself and my counseling staff, and Social Work.

Sometimes we talk about issues: "How are we going to deal with hallucinations?" or "How are we going to deal with depression?" or things like that. But oftentimes we'll talk specifically about people that we're seeing and how we can coordinate our approach to them so we're consistent, so they're not getting mixed messages. And I feel like we have an incredibly wonderful working relationship.

How have ministers and religious organizations fared during this epidemic?

I've helped at some of their trainings. The Interfaith Network—I've spoken at some of theirs, and MCC [Metropolitan Community Church]. I've been involved with some of them, either speaking at their trainings or else getting to know them here on the unit.

Now these are religious organizations that are pro-gay or that are, at least, not anti-gay, right?

Right. Dignity is a Catholic organization of gay men and lesbians. They've been amazing. They're wonderful. They have helped here a lot. They've been a wonderful resource when people want to talk to clergy.

Is that frequent?

It's not that frequent, but every once in a while it does come up. So we have some good resources in the community that we can use. We've had some problems. This is amazing, but we've had people of the fundamentalist, Moral-Majority type coming on the unit unannounced and uninvited and going into patients' rooms, and they'll get through six people's rooms, telling them that if they would just repent their evil ways, they could be cured, before we catch them!

It's been infuriating. I mean, they're so righteous and they lay such trips on people, and they're totally uninvited. So we've had to monitor and really try and screen people. We don't want to close the unit and lock the door and have people show an ID when they want to come in, but it's also frightening how people can get access to people and lay a trip on them that is just totally inappropriate.

We have had to screen some of the hospital chaplains because some of them are not open to gays. So primarily, if patients are asking for clergy or indicating that that's something they might want, we have some real good resources that we can get for them.

What's your impression of how the mainstream media has handled this?

(Laughs.) Well, lately, I'll tell you, I've stopped reading the papers. I have literally stopped watching television or reading the papers. I've gotten real frustrated with media. I think the media's improved a lot, but it seems like for a while there every—people are just irresponsible in the media, I think. People will print "This is the latest cure" without checking it out.

Are you speaking now of both gay and mainstream?

Uh-huh. I think it's true of both. I think that sensationalism sells papers, and that's what people print. They print sensationalism. If there's dirt on any organization, they print it, but they don't print the good work that the organization does. And what really infuriates me is that people that might need these services are only going to see this sensationalistic crap. It's a real injustice, not only to the organization—forget that—but the person that needs them. How would you make a decision if every organization is being attacked? Who would you know how to trust? So I get real angry at the fact that our whole media system is set up for sensationalism to make the news.

What about police services and fire services and toxic substance squads, and that sort of thing? What's your impression of how they have reacted?

Well, I don't know. I don't have all that much contact with them, so I don't feel like I know much at all about toxic substances. The police—we've had people from the Police Department come here and donate juices to the unit. They're as much individuals as anybody else. There are some people within the Police Department who are incredibly caring and concerned and wonderful people who want to help, who really want to help; and there are some who would, I think, just as soon turn their backs on it and ignore it or who have strong anti-gay feelings that are actually hostile. So I think it's made up out of people, once again.

How about the CDC and federal agencies? What is your impression of their response?

Well, for a while there when everybody was dragging their feet on the money, I was infuriated. I thought the message was anything but subtle: "Let 'em all die." In fact, it was literally stated by one senator [Helms]. So I feel like that's really frustrating and infuriating.

Probably I'm a left wing, I guess; I'm not very far over. I'm mostly middle of the road, but I'm much more human oriented, and building bombs and nuclear weapons while ignoring what's happening now makes me angry. I feel like we have a government where this isn't going to be a priority, and that makes me angry and frustrated.

Really, Reagan did veto the first request for funds.

Uh-huh. Right; I mean, it became loud and clear. Toxic shock and Legionnaires' disease get tremendous backing and financial support—because it's happening to legionnaires, you know, but we're talking about a lot more people, and because they're gay or because they're the IV-drug-use population, they are lumped as undesirable and "Let 'em die." I get real nervous when I think about what politicians can do with this and the levels to which they can carry it.

I don't think that people are totally without basis when they worry about, "Are gay men going to be put in concentration camps?" I think I can understand that fear. If we close baths, then what do we do next? We close the bars, then we close the whole gay community, and where does that kind of control end?

When they started talking about repealing the antiprejudice laws against gays in Texas, I said, "Jesus, you know, how can you? We're going to start repealing what people worked so hard for for all those years." So that kind of scares me—politicians.

How do you think the AIDS epidemic will influence society's treatment of homosexuals?

I had a lot of hope. I still have hope. I had a lot of hope at the beginning because of me getting to know gay men more, and becoming—I mean, I have gay friends that are as close as any friend I could ever hope to have, and will be my friends for a long time, whether AIDS exists or not. I feel like I've grown. My life's been richer for that. It's been a much richer experience, and my hope was that—when we were out there doing all this talking and there still was that going on—that people would also enrich their lives by opening to people that they didn't know as well, and that the communities would—there'd be more interaction, and that people would just start seeing everybody as people.

As humans, yeah.

As human, and that race, color, sexuality doesn't determine anything, really, about your human qualities, and I think it's a loss of a lot of people not to go beyond their community, their rigid boundaries about who they'll interact with. So I had a lot of hope that maybe in the midst of people dying, in the midst of all of this, the horribleness of this, that maybe there would be some good and that people would get to know other people and that we'd stop looking at stereotypes and we'd stop looking at people as if they're different from us, that we'd see that we're much more alike than different.

It doesn't sound like your hope has been sustained.

It's there, still, and it's hard to maintain it when there's so much infighting. There's so much craziness around that I hope that the good starts coming out and being seen as all the incredible stuff that is happening that's positive, and we can stop focusing on the negative. I know that I personally will come out of this a whole lot better a person. So I feel like I'm not going to lose anything.

As far as how big of a scope it's going to take, if it's going to end up just being in this city, if it's going to end up nationally, internationally, I don't know. Right now, at this moment—and this may change tomorrow—I feel discouraged about politicians and politicalness and divisiveness, and I hope that we can get beyond that.

In terms of the gay movement itself and the agenda for the gay movement, how do you think it should affect the agenda of the gay movement?

What should they be doing? They should be working together. I think that the politics needs to be decreased around this.

You mean the internal infighting?

The internal gay politics, you know, this Democratic club doesn't like that club and that—I mean, everybody's got their own agendas. You know, AIDS is a great bandwagon to step on in terms of getting some of your other agendas met, and I wish people could realize that that's not what's really needed.

The whole "Whitewash" article was real upsetting to me. I personally know how much the Public Health Department has done, and it's only because of people's politics that they're going to start attacking things. You know, Pat Norman started from a real caring, human place with the work for AIDS. I don't think it came from her self-motivation to get into a political position. But because that happened and she was getting into a political position, then the attacks came.

The people that really got hurt are the people doing the work here with people with AIDS, and the people with AIDS themselves. A few people who want political power or political recognition and the votes and the money are starting to get crazy at times.

How about the gay newspapers? Do you see that same kind of power?

Oh, for a long time it seemed there was a big fight between the *Sentinel* and the *B.A.R.*, and the *B.A.R.*'s real clear
that they're not behind Shanti and they're not behind any of
the organizations. They always print articles that are against
Shanti and against the AIDS Foundation without any editorial
note, but as soon as someone writes a letter in support, Paul
Lorch has to get in there and put some type of a comment on
it. So it's real clear where they're coming from.

**Why do you think they're coming from that kind of
space?**

Well, I think they're very sensationalistic oriented. I think
that that sells papers—attacking people sells papers. I think it's
incredibly poor journalism, first of all, to print an anonymous
letter as they did against Shanti. I think that's a poor statement
about their journalistic code of ethics, attacking someone else
by name in an anonymous letter. That seems pretty poor to
me.

Another thing, worrying about defending Shanti, I'm clear
that Shanti will go on through all this without being totally
destroyed by it at all, or even probably touched very much,
other than that it takes away our energy and it's undermining
and it would be nice to get support and not be attacked. And I
think it sells papers. The *Sentinel* has been sort of in our support more than the *B.A.R.* So the newspapers just want to
compete for themselves; it seems to me like that's their priority, and not truth.

So I think that the gay community has been amazing. I
mean, this unit here, we've gotten donations like you couldn't
believe, from everywhere. Chaps [a bar] has raised so much
money for 5B and for Shanti. At Christmastime they had a
Christmas tree there that they just strung lights on, and it cost
everybody five dollars to put a bulb on it and it was donated to

5B. And the tree lit up and they had to put a string of lights around the bar. Then we got these huge checks from them and they came in and catered this incredible dinner on Christmas Eve and Christmas Day.

On Tuesday night they catered food for the patients—the food here is terrible! And we've gotten pajamas and bathrobes and an interior decorating firm brought a Christmas tree in. The place looked like wonderland at Christmastime.

We've just gotten a tremendous amount of support from a lot of people in the gay community who quietly get out there and help and do the work, who aren't out for recognition, who really aren't out to get a position or whatever. There's been a tremendous amount of support coming from the gay community.

Let's talk for just a few minutes about male issues of power. A lot of the people that are coming down with AIDS are men, most of the people who are in positions of power and writing these newspapers are men. Do you see that as a real masculine trip?

I am not an authority on men and women. I have never been a political person, not even in the women's issues, so I have to claim no ability to make judgments. I do think that the outspokenness of people with AIDS—I don't know if they were women if they would have ever gotten as organized and been as assertive and as aggressive in making statements. I think that's true.

I think there's a quality about men in general being more assertive and more aggressive that has been helpful in the fact that the people with AIDS themselves have been able to say, "Hey," and have made themselves known. I think maybe that is a dynamic that does occur in politics that causes a lot of problems; that could be.

How do you think the AIDS epidemic will change the coming-out process itself? What's going to happen with the twelve-year-olds and the fourteen-year-olds today?

Twelve-year-olds and fourteen-year-olds, God! I would hate to be a gay man coming out right now. I would find it very hard to feel free to be expressive of my sexuality, at the same time confronting fear. I see parents grasping onto that even more. I think it would be incredibly difficult to come out now as a gay person and feel good and comfortable about it.

I think it's so hard now, with the judgments about being gay in our society, to develop a good sense of self-esteem and to see yourself as a valuable, wonderful, loving person. At the same time they're saying that being gay equals death, and is this my punishment? I feel sorry for any person right now trying to come out being gay or work through their own sexuality. I think it limits those choices.

Yeah, I think it limits people's choices, too. That's exactly what it does. Is there anything else that you would like to say?

I feel like it's an honor to be involved in this. I was on a straight board that voted for the project to take this direction, and it was an honor to be part of a straight board willing to recognize beyond their own, that there were no issues around limitations of people. I mean, people were people. I know that if this were sickle-cell anemia among blacks and blacks were dying, we would be there, too, and I feel really good that we've been able to do that.

I certainly hope it stops. It's become really hard here on the unit because we're just watching so many people die and it's not even just patients anymore, it's our friends. I've seen people at such a young age have to deal with issues that most of us never hope to deal with.

If people ever say to me that gay men are selfish or only interested in themselves and don't have any concern for anyone else, I'd have to tell them out-and-out that that's totally inaccurate, that I've seen so much love and so much caring. I was thinking the other day, if I died, would I have a community like this to support me? How wonderful and how horrible!

Why is there such a dichotomy of stuff around this? Like the horribleness of all these people dying and yet the wonderfulness of all the people that are helping and being there. It makes it sometimes impossible to understand.

I wish we could all be as loving as so many of the gay brothers have been to their friends dying—to everyone. There would be world peace.

Glossary

Alpha interferon: A new treatment for KS that involves the biological modification of the immune system. It is thought that this treatment does not destroy cells, but boosts a natural immune response.

Amebiasis: An infection with *Entamoeba histolytica*. Usually appears as an infection in the bowel but it can cause more generalized illness.

Burkitt's lymphoma: A malignant disease of the lymphoid tissue found among African children, caused by a virus or malarial infection and transmitted by biting insects.

CDC-defined AIDS: The Centers for Disease Control defines the surveillance definition of acquired immunodeficiency syndrome as the presence of reliably diagnosed disease at least moderately indicative of underlying cellular immunodeficiency such as Kaposi's sarcoma in a patient under sixty years old, *Pneumocystis carinii* pneumonia, or other opportunistic infections. These infections and diseases are in the absence of known causes of underlying immunodeficiency and of any other reduced resistency associated with the disease.

Cerebral dysfunction: A malfunction of the cortex, causing damage to motor control and mental functioning.

CMV (cytomegalovirus): CMV is a virus related to herpes. Infections may cause a range of symptoms from mild (flulike symptoms) to severe (pneumonia and hepatitis).

Flagyl: A drug used to treat amebiasis.

GRID (gay-related immune deficiency): The term for AIDS unofficially used before the introduction of the term Acquired Immune Deficiency Syndrome.

HTLV-III (human T-lymphotropic virus): The term coined in 1984 by the National Institute of Health to name a virus that looks like the LAV, and is present in some gay men who are now considered to have AIDS. At the time of this writing in late 1985 the HTLV classification is considered a misnomer, as the virus that causes AIDS is a *lente virus* (a slow-acting virus), not a T-lymphotropic virus.

Iatrogenic epidemic: An epidemic induced inadvertently by a physician or his treatment.

KS (Kaposi's sarcoma): Cancer of the walls of blood vessels. Usually seen on the surface of the skin, but death occurs from internal organ involvement that may be independent of the skin lesions. Classic KS has been distinguished from the more aggressive KS seen among gay men with AIDS, with classic KS being milder and involving skin primarily on extremities.

LAV (lymphadenopathy virus): The term coined in 1983 by the Institut Pasteur to name a virus discovered that might be the cause of disease underlying swollen lymph glands among gay men.

Lymphadenopathy: A swelling of the lymph glands found among gay men with AIDS; also present in conditions thought to be related to AIDS. Persistent and generalized swelling of the lymph glands may indicate infection with the AIDS virus, however, lymph glands sometimes swell in response to fighting *any* infection.

PCP (*Pneumocystis carinii* pneumonia): A lung disease that may indicate AIDS; caused by a common airborne protozoan. Among gay men with AIDS the survival rate after this infection may be up to eighteen months.

STDs: Sexually transmitted diseases are those diseases most commonly spread by sexual contact.

Thrush: An oral infection caused by *Candida albicans*, commonly known as a yeast infection.

Toxoplasmosis: A disease seen among gay men with AIDS; an opportunistic infection caused by the protozoan *Toxoplasma gondii*.

Visualization: Producing mental images that may be healing and relaxing to the individual. Cancer patients may "see" white cells attacking cancer cells, or envisage themselves as already well again.

VP-16 (Etoposide): A new experimental chemotherapy treatment used for KS.

About the Author

Lonnie Gene Nungesser was born in the Ozark Mountain region of southern Missouri, the second in a farming family of six children. He was licensed as a minister of the Southern Baptist Church at age seventeen and served as pastor for the Whetstone Baptist Church in Mountain Grove, Missouri. At the age of nineteen he moved to San Francisco, where he served as a patrolman for the United States Coast Guard; he received an honorable discharge and attended the College of Alameda for two years. In 1974 Nungesser was elected the first Caucasian student body president in this East Bay junior college; he successfully initiated a multiethnic and dual-gender system of self-government for the student body. He appeared in *Who's Who Among Students in American Technical and Vocational Schools* in 1975.

In the spring of 1979 Nungesser graduated from Stanford's Psychology Honors Program and was awarded one of the first national scholarships presented by the Gay Academic Union. Nungesser began his doctoral program at the State University of New York at Stony Brook in the fall of 1979. Upon completion of his Master's degree in 1982, Nungesser took temporary leave from academic study, and returned to California to complete *Homosexual Acts, Actors, and Identities*, published in 1983. He is currently conducting his doctoral research on chronic illness and quality of life with Professor Philip Zimbardo at Stanford University and Dr. Ronald Friend at Stony Brook.

This book may be kept

FOURTEEN DAYS

kept overtime.